WHEN NATURE NEEDS ASSIST
Medical Support with Active

Making Good Decisions

BRAIN: Benefits/ Risks / Alternatives/ Instinct/ Nothing

- **Benefits**? What info will be gained from this test? What effect will this treatment have? Why is it necessary now? How will it affect what we do next? How likely is it to work?
- **Risks** + side-effects? Physical + emotional/ to mother + baby? How likely to occur? How likely to lead to other interventions?
- **Alternatives**: Another way to get this info/ create this effect, which is not invasive?
- **Intuition/ instinct**: Does this feel right for us?
- **Nothing**: What if we wait / continue as we are? Agree a time to re-assess.

TIME to reflect...discuss...decide

YOUR BODY ~ YOUR BABY ~ YOUR CHOICE
Informed consent/ informed refusal

COMMUNICATION with partner, with medical carers (engage MW)
BIRTH PREFERENCES
DOULA www.doula.org.uk
Consultant Midwife, Senior/ Coordinating Midwife on shift

YOUR RIGHTS & RESOURCES ~ get good information at:
www.aims.org.uk   www.birthrights.org.uk   www.which.co.uk/birth-choice   www.nct.org.uk
www.sarawickham.com   www.sarahbuckley.com   www.nice.org.uk
Natural Caesarean birth plan at: www.activebirthcentre.com/blog

Successful Usage & Minimising Potential Harmful Effects

INDIVIDUALISED ASSESSMENT -not just policy/ routine

SELECTIVE USE: minimum DOSE & careful TIMING of interventions

ACTIVE BIRTH RESOURCES are still possible and beneficial:
SUPPORTED UPRIGHT POSITIONS for instinctive movement & deep rests
ENVIRONMENT for hormones... feel private, safe, dark, quiet, warm
SUPPORT... constant, compassionate, trusted companion
NOURISHMENT & REST
BREATH & AFFIRMATIONS

HEALING & RECOVERY- time, talking, privacy, nourishment, rest, skin2skin...

Jill Benjoya Miller/ ABC

WHEN NATURE NEEDS ASSISTANCE:
Medical Support with Active Birth

These are questions you might ask when considering if induction of labour is right for you and your baby, in order to get more individualised information. You can apply this example to any routine or intervention that you are being offered.

These questions are largely from midwife Sara Wickham and AIMS.

- Why do you feel I need to be induced?
- Am I or is my baby compromised or in imminent danger? If so, would a calm caesarean be safer?
- What are the benefits of being induced for my specific situation? How likely is it to be successful?
- What are the risks of being induced? How likely is it that these effects will happen? How likely is it that induction will lead to the need for further interventions?
- What is involved in induction?
- What % of women who are induced in this hospital end up having a caesarean or forceps/ventouse?
- What monitoring is available to me?
- Can I use the shower/ pool for pain relief?
- Can I go home in the early stages and come back to hospital at the times we agree upon?
- What are the alternatives to being induced? Including non-medical options. What are the benefits / risks of those?
- What if I leave it for a couple of days to think about?
- Please can you refer me to research/ evidence that supports your advice?
- Seek a second opinion, Supervisor of Midwives, AIMS, good resources?

Remember that guidelines are not rules, and they are not necessarily right for you. It is valuable to have full conversations with your medical carers, asking any questions. You can delay or decline induction, or seek further information to make your choice. You can also change your mind at any point during the process of decision-making.

Janet Balaskas' '6 Way' Breathing and Touch Relaxation

These are ways that women may naturally breathe in labour and while giving birth and are not 'techniques' as such. Usually women breathe in slowly through the nose, and exhale through the mouth or the nose. When practicing aim for the exhalation and inhalation to be more or less equal in length. Regular practice in combination with yoga practice will lead you to your own spontaneous way of breathing. Learning to focus on your breathing through the intensity of birthing is an invaluable tool. It can help you to go beyond pain as labour progresses, into the ecstatic state of consciousness that Mother Nature intends.

In Labour

- **Calm breathing** – practice during relaxation – useful in early labour and when resting between surges

- **Surge breathing** – belly breath – a deepening of calm breathing useful during surges – practice while relaxing, sitting up and in a variety of yoga postures and labour positions

- **Sound breathing** – useful during surges – they may lead you to your own spontaneous sounds

    Humming
    Ooh…oh…aah…
    Ommmm

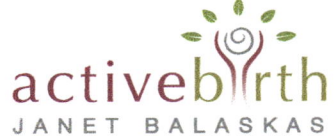

During Birth

Birth breathing – useful to 'breathe the baby down' along with the 'urge to push'. Practice these while leaning forward on all fours, over a ball or in the upright child position. Imagine a sense of downward pressure, which you will feel when the uterus tightens and pushes the baby down at this stage of the birth. Focus the breath 'down' through the centre of your body towards your pelvis and then further 'down' through the forward curve of the pevic canal as the baby's head moves down towards the perineum – 'the crowning'.

> Use the birth breathing with the <u>'slide visualization'</u>
> *Humming* – closed mouth with downward pressure towards the pelvis
> *Ooh...oh...aah...* spontaneous sound release

Light breathing – like gentle panting – useful at the end to slow down when the baby's head 'crowns' and with the <u>'opening rose visualization'</u>

Pressure breath – blowing on the first – useful in situations where more pressure is needed and more effort bearing down. This can also work well for a vaginal birth after epidural.

Massage and touch relaxation techniques

Anchors
- Shoulders
- Sacrum
- Hips
- Feet

Pressure point
- Sacrum (the natural epidural)
- Ankles

Light touch
- Arm
- Neck and shoulders
- 'Palm tree'

Full body strokes
- Standing
- Kneeling
- Sitting

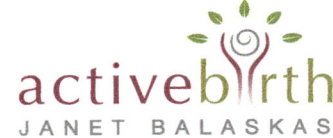

Affirmations for Active Birth

- My baby fits my pelvis perfectly

- My baby knows when to be born

- My body is softening and opening

- My body knows how to give birth

- My baby is moving down smoothly and easily

- My baby knows how to be born

- I can do this

- I am enjoying this

- I follow my breathing

- I soften all my muscles and relax

- I let go

- Giving birth is natural and safe

- I am ready to let go of my baby

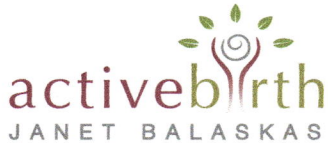

The Preparing for Labour and Birth Handbook

Information for informed decision making

This handbook was originally written for parents-to-be attending my Preparing for Labour and Birth courses. Over the years it became more comprehensive. The contents cover the definition and physiology of an active birth and also include information about complementary and medical back up that may be helpful, or necessary, during the different phases of labour and birth. It is an ideal companion to your ante-natal classes.

Giving birth is an instinct - it happens when your baby is ready to leave the womb. For the majority of women, labour has the potential to progress normally with no complications. You may not need any help other than the space and privacy to get on with it, the loving presence of your chosen companion and the motherly care of a skilled midwife.

However, birth is an unknown adventure and what will happen is unpredictable, so it's best to keep an open mind along with your dreams and strong intentions for your birth. If you need to combine active birth wisdom with medical intervention, then the information in this book will help you to minimise any potential for side effects, to stay in charge and to remain a confident and empowered participant in the birth of your baby.

So I offer this book to you and your birth partner. I recommend that you read it through and talk about the contents together. Then put the handbook aside and focus on the natural potential and power of your instincts.

I wish you and your baby a safe and happy birth.

With my best wishes,

Janet Balaskas

Janet Balaskas

Preparing for Active Birth Handbook
© Copyright Janet Balaskas 2001
Updated and reprinted 2004, 2006, 2007, 2015

Janet Balaskas asserts the moral right to be identified as the author of this work.

All rights reserved. No part of this publication may be reproduced, stored in a retrieval system, or transmitted, in any form or by any means, electronic, mechanical, photocopying, recording or otherwise, without the prior permission of the author.

Contents

What is an Active Birth?
- Active birthgiver rather than passive patient 1
- Much more than a matter of positions 4
- How to prepare for an active birth 4
- Beyond the birth 5
- Comparative benefits of an active birth .... 7 & 8

Wellbeing during labour
- Vaginal examinations 9
- Monitoring your baby's heartbeat 9
- Summary 12

Complementary therapies
- Homœopathy 13
- Homœopathy – Remedies for use in labour 14
- Aromatherapy 14
- Aromatherapy – Essential Oils for use in labour 15
- Transcutaneous electronic nerve stimulations (TENS) 15
- Maternity Reflexology 16
- Acupuncture 16

Medical pain relief
- Pethedine and Meptazenol 17
- Gas and Air (Entonox) 19
- Epidural Anaesthesia 20
- Spinal Anaesthesia 20
- Other forms of medical pain relief 24
- An alternative to medical pain relief – using a brth pool 24
- Guidelines for reducing and relieving pain in labour 26

Induction
- Premature and postmature babies 27
- What to do when you're overdue! 28
- Natural methods of inducing labour 30
- Medical methods of induction 31
- Accelerating labour 33
- Guidelines for medical induction 35
- The third stage controversy 36
- Guidelines for the use of Syntometrine 38

Assisting babies to be born
- Episiotomy 39
- Perineal massage 40
- Ventouse (vacuum extraction) or Forceps 43
- Caesarian section 46

Planning your birth (Creating your wish list) 49

Addendum – The Active Birth Manifesto

What is an Active Birth?

'First do nothing' - Hippocratic oath

Active birthgiver rather than passive patient

The question 'what is an active birth ?' can be answered on many levels.

Firstly, it means that there is a true partnership between you and your birth attendants, which encourages you to be an active participant in your pregnancy and birth rather than a passive patient. For this you need to be well informed about all your options. The Preparing for Labour and Birth Handbook covers the essential information you will need for empowered decision making for your birth. You will learn about normal birth physiology and how to enhance it with breathing, positions, massage, water and complementary therapies and also about medical interventions.

The emphasis with this approach is on having a wide range of choice which includes both holistic and medical options, and on your involvement, responsibility and control at all times, unless your choice is to leave the decision making to the professionals. This sense of partnership empowers you to be actively responsible and involved in all aspects of your care, so that your birth is an 'active birth' whether you manage it all naturally, opt for an epidural or have a caesarian. The birth is also viewed very much as part of the whole journey of becoming a parent which includes the emotional issues involved and anticipating what life will be like beyond the birth. This 'woman or family centred' approach is at the heart of Active Birth philosophy.

Your relationship with your midwives is another fundamental aspect of an Active Birth. Wherever possible you are encouraged to get to know them before the birth and to feel confident in their care. Traditionally, midwives are the primary attendants at a natural active birth and should have the skills and intuition to guide you and to create the best possible emotional and physical environment for a physiological birth. Many midwives are dedicated to empowering women to give birth normally, and you can request to be allocated a midwife who is experienced or supportive of Active Birth.

In the event of your needing medical help, the midwife's presence continues to support you alongside the doctor or obstetrician. It may not always be possible to meet the midwives who will be attending you in labour in advance. If this is the case. then try to meet the senior midwife of your team and it is a good idea to write a 'wish list' to attach to your notes. (see page 49)

The environment for an active birth

In an active birth the normal physiological processes are enabled, as much as possible, to unfold without disturbance. The aim is to provide the optimal environment and to let labour progress naturally in its own time and rhythm. While most births can be expected to progress normally, there is also the reassuring awareness that medical pain relief or interventions can be considered at any time, should the need arise.

Labour and birth are involuntary, in that the uterus contracts spontaneously, firstly to open the womb and then to give birth to the baby. All of this happens without our conscious control. We can understand the importance of the environment when we ask the question 'what makes labour happen?' From beginning to end the entire process is stimulated by hormones produced by the mother's 'old brain' or hypothalamus. We have this in common with all other mammals, and like them, we need to feel safe and protected in order to secrete the birth hormones effectively. These are the very same hormones we produce when we make love, which is why the pioneering French obstetrician Michel Odent calls them the 'love hormones'. Think about the kind of environment you like to be in when you make love, or how mammals usually choose a warm dark and secure place to give birth and you can guess what kind of atmosphere will encourage good secretion of these 'love hormones' during labour. [1]

The optimal environment for an active birth will feel comfortable, warm, safe and familiar, allowing you a real feeling of privacy. The midwife will give motherly support and offer unobtrusive and sensitive care. You are

---

1   Odent, M. *Why labouring women don't need support.* Mothering Magazine. Autumn 1996, pp. 46-50

free to move, breathe, change positions, use a birth pool, make as much noise as you need to, have your own music, dim the lights, use aromatherapy and homoeopathy (see pages 14 and 15) and have the support of the birth partner/s of your choice. This kind of relaxed and calm atmosphere encourages the secretion of hormones such as oxytocin, which stimulates uterine contractions, and endorphines, which are like natural relaxants and pain relievers. This means that labour progresses well and your body's natural chemistry helps you to cope with the pain. These hormones also promote 'attachment' behaviour. The high level of hormones in mother and baby after a physiological birth ensure that they fall in love, or 'bond' immediately after the birth.[2]   A homelike, hormone enhancing environment, where you can relax and let go without inhibition to the power of the birth process is essential for an active birth. For many women, having a home birth is the best way to create the perfect environment for birthing. For others, the added security of obstetric support on the premises, makes a birth centre or hospital which encourages physiological birth, the best choice.

Instinct and intuition

Your body is ideally designed to birth a baby and inherently knows what to do.

Given freedom and privacy in labour, you will probably follow your instincts and want to move your body and change positions to make yourself as comfortable as possible during contractions and while resting inbetween them. At its most practical level, an active birth involves having the freedom to use upright positions such as standing, walking, kneeling or squatting. You will need some simple props such as a beanbag, low stool or birth ball so that you can be comfortably supported in these 'gravity effective' positions. This means that you are free to be led by your own powerful intuition, to move spontaneously and to guide your baby down through the birth canal in the most effective way.

You will also be doing what women all over the world have done for thousands of years. Active birth has been the norm in every culture on earth since time immemorial. It was only 300 years ago in the 17th century that forceps were invented and women began to lie down for birth in the 'stranded beetle' position. The birth of obstetrics in Europe at that time led to the marvellous obstetric 'safety net' we have all over the developed world today. However, along the way birth became over medicalised and age old birth wisdom and midwifery skills were lost. Today active birth is being rediscovered and we have the benefit of modern obstetrics too, so that whatever you want or need for your birth should usually be attainable.

Using upright positions has many benefits

- The baby naturally aligns itself in the best possible position with the help of the downward force of gravity. Your intuitive movements in these positions will help your baby to be born.

- Gravity ensures that the baby's head is well applied to the cervix so contractions are more effective which may result in faster dilation and a shorter labour.

- Freedom of movement, free expression of sound and the natural forward tilting of the uterus helps to modify the pain and may reduce the need for an epidural if you prefer not to have one.

- The pelvic joints are unconstricted as they would be lying down and this allows a degree of movement and expansion of the pelvic diameters so that the internal shape of the pelvis can accommodate the baby's head with maximal space as it descends in labour. In the final stages, the back wall of the pelvis (sacrum and coccyx) are free to move back increasing the diameters of the pelvic outlet to make plenty of space for your baby to make his or her way down and out.

- Blood flow to the placenta is optimal in upright positions. There is no compression of the internal blood vessels as there may be if you lie for an extended period on your back or in the semi-reclining position. This ensures that your baby has enough oxygen throughout and reduces the risk of foetal distress.

- In the second stage it is much more effective and powerful to push with the help of gravity and the baby's rotation and descent through the birth canal is easiest.

---

2   Odent, M. *The Scientification of Love*. Free Association Press. London 1999.

- Gravity also helps the safe separation of the placenta once your baby is born and sitting upright will help you to hold your baby in a good position as you welcome your baby and help him or her to breastfeed for the first time.

- Partners are often actively involved in giving both emotional and physical support. This sharing of the birth experience can be very fulfilling and memorable and is a good start to a new relationship and a new family.

- At the end of the day you are likely to feel exhilarated and empowered by the whole experience. You will have a very high level of oxytocin, the hormone that makes you fall in love with your baby forever!

How do babies benefit from an active birth?

- Good oxygenation of the blood supply to the placenta in upright positions and the easiest possible angle of descent through the pelvis reduce the risk of foetal distress.

- There are fewer side effects from drugs or interventions.

- Labour and birth are potentially quicker and usually uncomplicated, so there is minimal trauma for the baby and a positive start in life.

- The baby is likely to be born in optimal condition.

- Bonding after birth and the first breastfeeding are facilitated and the mother generally feels good and recovers well from the birth, which makes caring for the newborn baby easier.

Using a birth pool

Besides gravity, water is another of nature's elements which has enormous power to support and encourage the birth process. In mid labour (when you are about 5-6 cms dilated) can be a good time to think of entering the birth pool. The warm sensations of the water on your skin help to modify the pain and the buoyancy of the water supports your body's weight. This helps enormously to make you more comfortable in upright positions and to conserve your strength and energy. It's much easier for most women, for example, to squat in water than it is on land. Your partner can sit right beside the pool or even get in with you to massage and hold you.

There is an increase in oxytocin secretion when you enter the water which peaks after about 2 hours, so you may find that contractions become stronger and you reach full dilation within a few hours. (Although this is often the case, it may not work like that for everyone.) [3]

Once in the pool, you are unlikely to notice how much time has passed as this soothing environment helps you to go so deeply inside yourself that you are completely relaxed and surrendered to the involuntary rhythms of your labour. If at any time contractions slow down in the pool, then it is best to get out and use the help of gravity on dry land.

When you feel you are ready to push and give birth to your baby you may decide to leave the pool and have your feet firmly planted on the ground or you may decide to remain in the water for the second stage. When progress is good, birth in water is safe and gentle for the baby, so it is a popular option with midwives or hospitals that have experience of this style of birthing. Reliable portable water birth pools with firm sides can be hired from a number of companies. Links to these companies can be found on the Active Birth Centre website which is www.activebirthcentre.com.

---

3   Odent, M. *Can water immersion stop labour?* Journal of Nurse-Midwifery, vol 42, No 5. September/October 1997, pp 414-416.

Much more than a matter of positions

Being pregnant, giving birth and becoming a parent are profound experiences. Understanding what happens to you emotionally throughout the entire transition is another important aspect of an active birth. In the active birth yoga classes during your pregnancy, you will be encouraged to get in touch with your feelings and to give time and focus to your 'inner world'. There are also many opportunities to talk with Active Birth teachers, complementary therapists, midwives and obstetricians. While they may not be able to solve your problems, having someone who understands, to listen to you and to talk with, is an enormous help in getting through the challenges that arise at this time in your life. Sometimes one -to -one counselling can be very positive and productive if the emotional challenges seem overwhelming. The involvement and support of partners is often invaluable and they are encouraged to participate in all aspects of an active birth. If you are a single parent, it is possible to create an alternative support system and to involve a partner of your choice as well.

The birth of a family is the essence of an active birth. Families today have different shapes and sizes and everyone is involved in welcoming the new baby. During your journey into parenthood, a fetus becomes a baby, a woman becomes a mother, a man becomes a father, children become brothers and sisters and everyone involved becomes a family. The birth itself is only one event, albeit an important one, in the whole adventure.

The early weeks and months after your baby is born are usually very challenging and few people anticipate how much life will change. Active birth is about maintaining the continuum from pregnancy into parenting in the smoothest possible way. The aim of an active birth is a successful transition into 'active parenting.' The Active Birth Centre and our nationwide network of teachers are renowned for giving integrated support to the family as a whole, which continues beyond the birth into the postnatal period.

Our post natal programme offers support and advice on all aspects of life after birth. Baby massage classes help you to enhance your relationship with your baby through the powerful language of touch and post natal yoga restores your energy. As well as the company of other new parents at these sessions and continued contact with the teachers, there are also special events on parenting, homoeopathy, vaccination issues, resuscitation of babies and first aid, and a specialised complementary therapies and well baby clinic. You are encouraged to visit the weekly 'mothers talking' sessions before and after you have your baby as often as you can, or to join a local support group. That way you get the chance to talk to new parents and make new friends, see plenty of babies and maybe get to hold one or two, observe breastfeeding and bottle feeding, check out what equipment seems most useful, see how nappies are changed and to learn about the reality of life beyond the birth!

How to prepare for an active birth

In addition to the 'Preparing for Labour and Birth' course, Active and Water Birth workshops, Yoga for Pregnancy is a vital part of your inspiration and preparation for an active birth. These sessions are held throughout the week at the Active Birth Centre. You can join at any time and you are encouraged to attend weekly throughout your pregnancy, if possible. There are teachers trained at the Active Birth Centre in many other parts of London and the UK and a list of teachers can be obtained from our website "contact" menu at www.activebirthcentre.com. Books, CD's and tapes for self practice are available by mail order.

What kind of yoga?

The approach is gentle, yet powerful and based on a unique style of yoga which combines traditional Hatha Yoga with postural principles which are similar to the Alexander technique. This approach to yoga was pioneered by Vanda Scaravelli, a renowned and innovative yoga teacher from Italy. The yoga taught in the classes is especially modified to accommodate the physical, emotional and physiological changes of pregnancy. As it avoids strain or pushing yourself beyond your comfortable limit, it is ideal for this time and is suitable for anyone, whether you are a total beginner or an experienced practitioner. The emphasis is on slow, thoughtful practise of simple postures which can be easily adapted to everyone's comfort, combined with meditative awareness of the wavelike rhythm of the breath. You are encouraged to discover your body's relationship with the downward force of gravity and to experience the release of tension, lightness and freedom of the spine which follows. You will leave every class more comfortable with yourself, more relaxed, with more space in your body for your baby and for your breathing, and a growing sense of confidence.

Breathing awareness and meditation

The concentration on your spontaneous breathing rhythm which you will learn in these classes is invaluable practise for labour. You will find that you can use this 'inner focus' during contractions and mentally channel the power of the breath to release pain. Body memory gained in the classes returns instinctively in labour, so that there is no need to learn any breathing techniques. Even during caesarean section with epidural, this ability to relax and focus on your breath is very calming and useful. This can be an amazing tool, no matter what happens. To be really effective, practise is needed in pregnancy by coming regularly to the class and/or practising on your own at home.

The direct benefit of yoga in pregnancy is the relaxation, time and focus you are able to give to yourself and your baby. Women find the yoga an oasis of calm which helps to make their pregnancy more enjoyable and also more healthy. In addition to 'de-stressing', you will be able to find that slow, quiet time every pregnant woman and new mother needs. This will help you to 'bond' with your baby on a deeper level long before the actual birth and to reduce fatigue afterwards. It will also give you the peace and space to be in touch with your deepest feelings, your instincts and intuition. In this sense it is profoundly empowering.

How your body benefits

The more obvious physical benefits are better breathing and circulation, well toned pelvic floor muscles, increased flexibility and improved posture. The yoga classes include a lot of focus on the way you walk, stand, sit and kneel which can be applied to your everyday activities. Good posture also helps to avoid or alleviate pain in the sacro-iliac joints, back pain and pubic pain.

Of course when your own posture is balanced there is the added benefit of naturally carrying and positioning your baby well. Jean Sutton, a renowned New Zealand midwife, calls this 'optimal foetal positioning' and there are plenty of tips in the classes about how to use your body to increase the chances of your baby settling into the best position for birth. This awareness extends into labour and develops your intuitive sense of how to move positively to enhance the progress of labour and birth. [4]

Labour and birth positions

Learning useful labour positions with your body during these sessions will awaken your instincts and your innate ability to cope with labour and birth, just as millions of women have done before you! Yoga also helps you to make the most of your body's natural increase in flexibility in pregnancy to become more comfortable in upright positions you may want to use for the birth. You will be shown, for example, how to become more at ease in supported squatting positions which open the pelvis to its widest. This will make it easier to give birth to your baby and can even be used to give birth after an epidural.

Beyond the birth

Most women who have an active birth feel very pleased, satisfied and proud of themselves whether it was a physiological birth or not, and recover very quickly. At the end of the day it is a great achievement to bring a healthy new baby into the world, however it needs to happen. However, if the birth was far more difficult than anticipated, or there were complications, some women feel disappointed that reality did not meet their expectations. Sometimes it is beyond our power to influence the progress or outcome of the birth. When this happens, feeling some disappointment is fair enough and you will need to go through those natural feelings; however this should not go on too long and generally the excitement and challenge of looking after your new baby will soon put these feelings behind you. Occasionally when this is not the case, some counselling or debriefing may be needed to come to terms with what happened. Your Active Birth teacher should be able to do this with you or put you in touch with a therapist or counsellor.

In pregnancy the active birth approach is to encourage you to keep an open mind as well as a strong intention. Birth is unpredictable and its always best to keep your priorities in perspective. Never let your own experience of birth become more important than the wellbeing of your baby. At the end of the day what matters most to all of us is the safety and wellbeing of mother and baby. If your birth is difficult, your birth attendants can try their best to maintain the spirit of an active birth and may advise medical care if necessary, sometimes in combination with supported upright positions.

---

4   Sutton, J. and Scott, P. *Understanding and teaching Optimal Foetal Positioning*. Birth Concepts. New Zealand. 1996.

After your birth you will find that the ability to centre and ground yourself that you learnt from your yoga practise and the ability to release tension with breathing awareness is an empowering tool for life. Many of the movements and postures are applicable after the birth to release tension from your back, neck and shoulders after carrying your baby and to relax deeply in the brief intervals of solitude that you will get as a new mother. Postural awareness is also vital in the early months and years when your child needs to be lifted and carried regularly.

Perhaps the greatest benefit of attending a pregnancy yoga class is the supportive and informative company of the other women in the group. Partner work and massage is part of the class and women enjoy and appreciate this work with touch and contact with others going through the same transition. You get to hear lots of birth stories after the class and to meet some very young babies, when class members return for a visit after the birth. Many long term friendships have their origins in pregnancy yoga classes.

If you don't live near to the Active Birth Centre or a local teacher, don't despair. Our books and tapes are very helpful and many women find them useful and effective preparation for birth. I especially recommend my book 'Preparing for Birth with Yoga' and the double CD, booklet and wallchart 'Yoga for Pregnancy'.

Join the Active Birth E-Journal

I'd like to invite you to prepare for your birth online by subscribing to my e-journal which is sent out fortnightly by email. You will receive 5 or 6 very helpful articles from 12 weeks of pregnancy until your baby is 6 months old. To join, go to **www.activebirthcentre.com** and subscribe on the home page.

The Comparative Benefits of an Active Birth

UPRIGHT POSITIONS

Squatting, standing, kneeling

Gravity Effective

Weight of baby's head and body puts even pressure from above on cervix and results in faster dilation.

Uterus tilts forward during contractions

With the mother leaning forward this can happen without resistance so contractions work more efficiently with less pain.

No weight on major blood vessels

Leaning forward allows better blood flow to baby and placenta, and better oxygenation so there is less risk of foetal distress.

Sacrum mobile

Pelvic canal can widen and adjust to the shape of the baby's descending head.

Pelvic joints can expand

Less pressure on joints reduces pain (especially back ache). More space as internal pelvic proportions increase.

RECLINING POSITIONS

Supine, semi-reclining

Oppose gravity

Less pressure on the cervix from baby's weight. Uneven pressure on cervix results in slower dilation and more likelihood of an anterior lip.

Uterus works against gravity

These positions oppose gravity, and the resulting resistance make contractions less efficient and more painful.

Weight of uterus compresses major blood vessels

Can compromise blood flow to the uterus increasing the risk of foetal distress.

Sacrum immobile

With the mother's body weight resting on the sacrum, the pelvic outlet is narrowed.

Pelvis less mobile

More pressure on nerves increases perception of pain. Less space for baby as internal proportions of pelvis decrease.

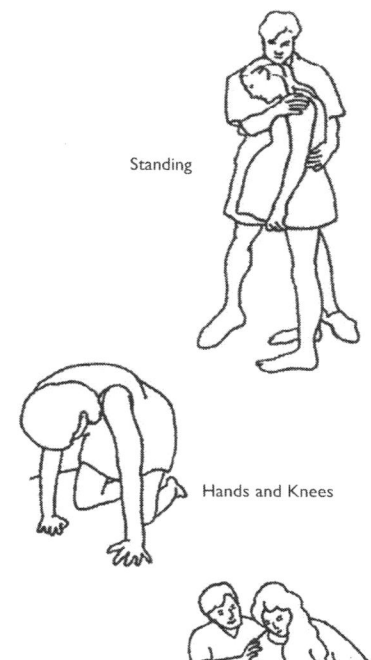
Standing

Hands and Knees

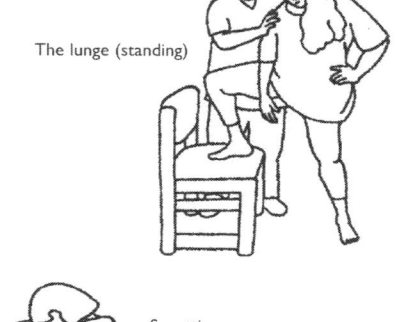
The lunge (standing)

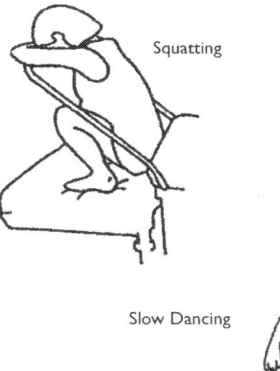
Squatting

Slow Dancing

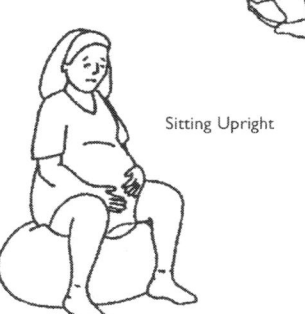
Sitting Upright

Second stage - pelvis upright

Baby's angle of descent is easiest - down and out.

Uterus can exert maximum force making bearing down more efficient and shortening the second stage.

Perineum expands evenly

Reduces the risk of tearing.

Baby at birth in optimal condition when birth is active

Less need for painkillers or interventions reduces risk of side effects. Mother feels proud, empowered and satisfied.

Remaining upright for third stage

- Gravity assists separation and expulsion of the placenta and retraction of the uterus, reducing the need for Syntometrine.

- Fluids drain effectively from uterus, reducing risk of infection.

- Easy to position the baby well for first sucking. Latching on to breast stimulates uterus to contract and reduces blood loss.

Second stage - pelvis horizontal

Baby's angle of descent is more difficult - up hill.

Bearing down force made less efficient, prolonging second stage.

Perineum cannot expand evenly

Baby's head presses directly on the perineum and risk of tearing increases.

Baby at birth may be compromised when birth is passive

Greater need for painkillers or interventions with possible side effects.

Lying down after birth

- Less efficient separation and expulsion of placenta. Slower retraction of the uterus may create need for Syntometrine to prevent excessive blood loss.

- Fluids tend to pool in the uterus, increasing risk of infection.

- More difficult to position baby well for breastfeeding.

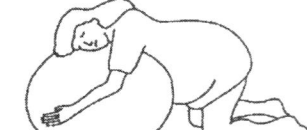
Kneeling over birth ball

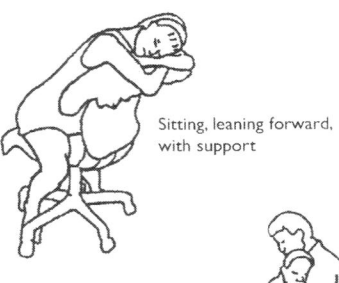
Sitting, leaning forward, with support

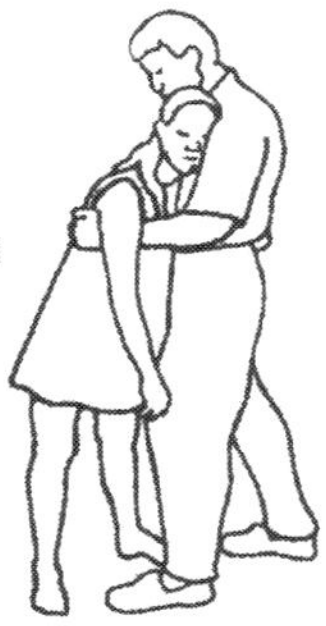

Standing, leaning forward

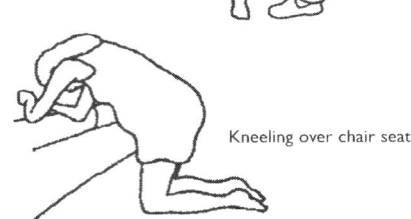
Kneeling over chair seat

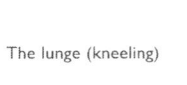
The lunge (kneeling)

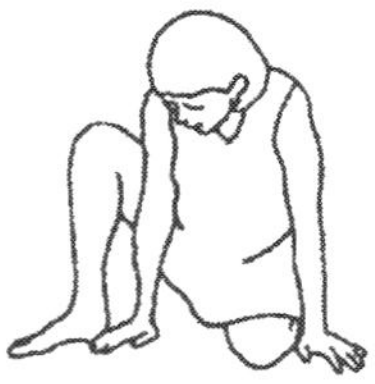

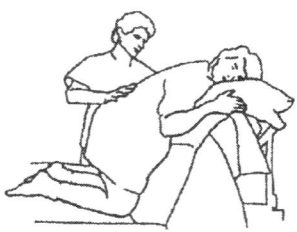
Kneeling, leaning on raised head of bed

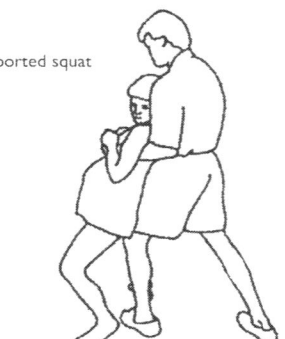
Supported squat

- Drawings by Shanna Dela Cruz, copyright Ruth Ancheta 1994 and 1999 from 'the Labor Progress Handbook', Blackwell Science, Oxford 2000.
- Recommended reading: New Active Birth by Janet Balaskas, Thorsons, London 1991.

Wellbeing During Labour

During labour your midwife will be checking your progress regularly as well as making sure that you and your baby are doing well. At the first check she will ask you how you are and what's been happening, measure your blood pressure, take your body temperature and test a sample of your urine. These basic checks on your well-being may be repeated periodically. She will also check the lie and position of your baby by feeling your abdomen, and may perform an internal vaginal examination to assess how far your cervix has dilated. Throughout labour your baby's heartbeat will be checked at regular intervals to ensure that he or she is coping well and that there is no sign of foetal distress.

Vaginal examinations

Vaginal examinations, or VEs, are done by the midwife, with your permission, to assess the softness, thickness, position and dilation of the cervix. She will wear disposable latex gloves and use a lubricant and then insert two fingers into the vagina so that she can feel the cervix. Once the cervix has dilated sufficiently, she will also be able to feel the top of the baby's head. The position of the fontanelle (soft spot) will help her to assess the position of the presenting head.

Vaginal examinations are routinely done every four hours, at your request, or at the midwife's discretion. When labour progresses well they are often not needed at all. It is important to request a VE immediately before an intervention such as an epidural so that you know how dilated you are (see Medical Pain Relief, p.17). If you don't want to know how far you have dilated, you can ask the midwife not to tell you.

The midwife usually inserts her hand gently into the vagina immediately after a contraction and may complete the examination before the next one, or pause and continue once it is over.

It is not usually necessary for you to lie down as the VE can be done in a variety of positions, such as kneeling on all fours, sitting upright on the edge of a chair, in a water pool, or standing with one foot on a stool or chair. Discuss these possibilities with your midwife in advance. Let the midwife know when you are ready for her to start, then relax and breathe deeply – this will prevent unnecessary discomfort. Internal examinations can feel intrusive or painful and increase the risk of infection if the membranes are leaking or have ruptured. Some midwives believe that routine VE's are outmoded practise.[1]

Monitoring your baby's heartbeat

Your midwife will also be making sure that your baby is coping well with labour by checking your baby's heartbeat periodically. The first reading will form the baseline for comparison throughout labour. If the rhythm of the baby's heart changes significantly it is a possible indication of foetal distress and may mean that your baby needs some help. It is normal for the heartbeat to slow down a little immediately after a contraction. This natural deceleration means that the midwife needs to listen to the baby's heart both during and in between the contractions to get an accurate reading. Monitoring is usually done two or three times an hour in labour, and more frequently in the second stage if necessary. Continuous monitoring is only necessary when interventions are being used or if there is some concern about the baby's condition.

It is not necessary to lie on your back while you are being monitored. It may be much more comfortable to kneel on all fours, kneel upright, over a beanbag or birth ball, or sit on the edge of a chair. Monitoring is also easy to do under water in a birth pool in any of the above positions using a waterproof doptone, or by floating up and raising your pelvis close to the surface, or sitting up on the rim. Breathing and relaxing and 'saying hello' to your baby while being monitored will help to minimise disturbance.

There are several different ways that the foetal heart can be monitored and it is advisable to find out what method your birth attendants usually use. You can ask to see what the heart monitors look like and how they are used.

---

1 Warren, C. *Why should I do vaginal examinations?* The Practising Midwife. June 1999. Vol 2, No 6. pp 12-13

Intermittent monitoring

Intermittent monitoring is suitable for a normal, uncomplicated labour, and is done from time to time rather than continuously. There are several methods which can be used:

- **Ear trumpet or pinard**

    This is applied to your abdomen using sufficient pressure to obtain a reading. The midwife counts the number of heartbeats per minute. It is completely harmless and possibly a bit uncomfortable, as the midwife needs to press the trumpet quite firmly against your abdomen.

- **Doctor's stethoscope**

    An ordinary doctor's stethoscope can be used instead of a pinard. This is easier to use in upright positions.

- **Hand-held electronic monitor (Doptone or Sonic Aid)**

    This works by using ultrasound waves. The sound of the heartbeat is magnified and can be heard in the room. There are small portable versions which can be used in the home, and larger ones in hospitals which also produce a graphic printout of the heartbeat rhythms and the contractions. Waterproof hand-held monitors can also be used under water.

    The transducer is held against the mother's abdomen on the spot closest to the baby's heart. A lubricant may be used. The method is painless but some pressure may be needed to get a clear reading, and this is also the case with a pinard or stethoscope.

    Hand-held monitors are very convenient and easy to use for an active birth. Some women prefer not to expose their babies to even the mild doses of ultrasound used by these monitors. There is no evidence to suggest that this is harmful but, equally, there is no evidence yet available to assure us of long-term safety either.[2]

- **Continuous foetal heart monitoring**

    Continuous monitoring may be appropriate when interventions such as epidurals or inductions are being used, or when there is concern about the baby's condition.

- **Abdominal belt monitor**

    First the pulse rate may be recorded. Then belts or an elasticated band are placed on the mother's abdomen to hold the transducer in place. There are also newer versions which attach with suction pads. Sometimes two transducers are used, one to measure the baby's heartbeat and one to measure the contractions. This is known as cardiotocographic monitoring (or CTG), which produces a graph record of the foetal heartbeat and the duration and strength of the contractions. These involve the use of ultrasound, similar to a doptone but held in position continually by the belt.

    Most hospitals like to do a period of continuous CTG monitoring for 20-30 minutes or so as a routine when you first arrive, and may wish to repeat this periodically later in labour. There is no evidence that either of these procedures is of any value. While some women do not mind this, others find it disruptive and uncomfortable. This form of monitoring can be used while you are standing, sitting on a chair or kneeling, provided your movements do not cause the monitor to slip and interrupt the trace. This form of monitoring also uses ultrasound.

    Advantages:

    - Continuous monitoring with an abdominal belt can be very reassuring when interventions are being used or the baby is at risk.
    - It is non-invasive, although it may be uncomfortable to wear the belt. The transducers are simply held in position externally on the mother's abdomen.

    Disadvantages:

    - False readings can occur if the machinery is faulty or the interpretation of the readings is poor. Sometimes this can be the cause of unnecessary interventions.

---

2   More information about ultrasound can be obtained from the Association for Improvements in the Maternity Services, London.

- If the machine breaks down unexpectedly, it may cause unnecessary panic about the baby's condition.
- TENS (see pg 15) interferes with electronic monitoring and cannot be used simultaneously.
- Continuous monitoring that relies on a machine can become a substitute for personal care in a busy labour ward.
- Belt monitoring can confine the mother to a semi-reclining position and thus increase the risk of foetal distress. Full mobility is difficult although it is possible to use sitting, kneeling or standing positions. Some women find the belts uncomfortable, making it more difficult to cope with the pain of labour.

- ## Scalp electrode

    When babies are thought to be at risk, this form of monitoring may be used. An electrode is attached to the baby's head through the dilating cervix. The membranes need to be ruptured in order to attach the electrode. It may be possible to sit on a birth stool or use some upright positions with this kind of monitoring. Monitoring with a scalp electrode is not necessary for a normal labour.

    Advantages:

    - Considered to be the most accurate form of monitoring.
    - Can be reassuring when there is concern about the baby's well-being.
    - Greater mobility may be possible compared to being attached to a belt monitor if the flex is long enough, and birth attendants are encouraging.
    - A sample of the baby's blood can be obtained from the scalp to help assess the oxygen levels accurately and confirm the scalp electrode reading.

    Disadvantages:

    - The rupture of membranes, which must be done prior to attaching the scalp electrode, increases the risk of infection and pressure on the baby's head during second stage. It will also increase the intensity of the contractions which are likely to become stronger and more painful quite suddenly (see ARM on page 33, Induction)
    - This is an invasive form of monitoring for both mother and baby.
    - Some babies suffer a minor wound to the scalp which may leave a bald spot later on. Application of the monitor to the scalp may be painful for the baby and increases the risk of any potential infection from mother to baby if an infection is already present in the vagina (eg group B Strep)
    - Full mobility for the mother is not possible in case the electrode should become dislodged.
    - When used routinely for normal labours, studies from all over the world have shown conclusively that this form of monitoring increases the number of caesarean sections.[3]

- ## Telemetry

    Used in conjunction with the scalp electrode or alternatively, in some places, with an abdominal transducer, this transmits the baby's heart rate by radio waves and makes freedom of movement more possible for the mother as she is connected to a machine by a flex. It is still necessary to rupture the membranes prior to attaching the electrode if this method is used and the risks of doing this still apply. The equipment is not available in all hospitals.

---

[3] Murphy K., Johnson P., Pattison R., Russell V and Turnbull A. (1990) *Birth Asphyxia and the intrapartum cardiotograph.* British Journal of Obstetric Gynaecology, 97: 470-479.

Summary

Vaginal examinations

- Assess the dilation and thickness of the cervix.
- Assess the position of the baby's head or presenting part.
- May not be needed at all in a normal labour with good progress.
- May be done four hourly, in accordance with hospital protocols, at the midwife's discretion or the mother's request.
- Should always be done immediately before using interventions so you know how far dilated you are and can choose the appropriate form of pain relief or other intervention.

Monitoring the baby's heart beat

When labour is normal the following methods may be used:

- Ear trumpet or pinard.
- Stethoscope
- Hand held Doptone or Sonicaid

If the baby is at risk or if interventions are used:

- Hand held Sonicaid used frequently
- Continuous belt (CTG) monitoring
- Continuous monitoring by scalp electrode

Complementary Therapies

Complementary therapies can be very helpful in labour, and will enhance the natural process and modify pain without side effects when used appropriately. Homœopathy, aromatherapy and TENS have been selected for this booklet as they can be used very easily in labour and are usually effective. The remedies and oils recommended here are compatible and can be used simultaneously. If you already use acupuncture, acupressure, cranial osteopathy or herbs, you may use them safely in labour under the guidance of a trained therapist. Generally, it is best not to combine herbs with homœopathy unless with the help of a skilled practitioner.

Homœopathy

Homœopathic remedies can be invaluable during labour and can enhance the physiological process without any harmful side effects. While not within the scope of this information to explain the principles of homœopathy, we recommend further reading or consulting a homœopath during pregnancy for specific advice relating to labour.

To find out more, you can visit the shopping pages on our website to purchase a special kit of remedies for childbirth with comprehensive instructions. If you live locally, you can visit our homœopathic drop in clinic at the Active Birth Centre. A homœopathic pharmacy which supplies individual remedies by mail order is listed overleaf.

Remedies in the 200th potency are generally recommended for use in labour when symptoms are intense. They are best ordered as soft tablets or pillules that dissolve quickly in the mouth.

Homœopathic remedies are delicate. Touch them as little as possible. Shake one pill into the lid of the phial and tip it into the palm of the person taking the remedy, who should put it directly into their mouth. Remedies should be allowed to dissolve in a clean mouth and do not need to be taken with water or food. Discard any remedies that fall out accidentally. Store your remedies in a cool, dark, dry place.

The remedies listed in the table on the next page are recommended for general use during labour. They can be used to support the natural birth process or alongside other medication or interventions. Homœopathic remedies can also speed healing and recovery after the birth. Unless you get the kit, it's a good idea to label individual remedies beforehand according to their use, eg. 'pain', 'backache', 'weepy' etc. It usually works best if the birth partner or attendant takes responsibility for offering the woman any remedies that she needs so that she can concentrate on her labour. Observe her physical and emotional state carefully and offer her the remedy which seems most appropriate. If she does not seem interested, she does not need a remedy at that time. Try to avoid disturbing the rhythm of labour and offer her the remedy between contractions when she "emerges" and makes contact with you herself.

It's best to use only one remedy at a time and repeat only if the symptoms return. If the remedy does not seem to help, then try a different one. If she is showing more than one relevant symptom, e.g. if she is in pain (Arnica) and exhausted (Kali Phos), then allow ten minutes or so between remedies.

Generally, remedies can be given at half hourly intervals but can be taken at shorter intervals if symptoms are acute, or longer intervals if symptoms improve. When using homœopathy for pain relief, it is advisable to begin early on when she first begins to find contractions painful.

HOMOEOPATHY - REMEDIES FOR USE IN LABOUR

Arnica 200	This wonderful remedy is beneficial to most women in labour. It can be administered regularly throughout labour to help the muscles function properly, and to reduce exhaustion and pain.	Label as **Pain I**
Aconite 200	Reduces fear, anxiety and panic. It is very helpful where labour is too fast and the woman is frightened by this, or where contractions are overwhelming. Can be taken before labour where there is fear or anxiety about the birth.	Label as **fear**
Bellis Perrenis 200	Useful for deep abdominal pain where Arnica is not working	Label as **pain** II
Caullophyllum 200	Used to promote strong productive contractions in early labour. Useful where contractions are ineffectual, sharp, painful, and short, often concentrated in the lower abdomen and groin. Also good for weak contractions due to exhaustion in a long labour. Do not use routinely throughout labour.	Label as **weak contractions I**
Gelsemium 200	Next best choice if Caullophyllum doesn't help with weak contractions. Presents with physical heaviness, heavy eyes and limbs. Muscular weakness leading to trembling, chilliness and the 'stage fright' of transition. Also a great remedy to use if there is an anterior lip.	Label as **weakness and transitional exhaustion**
Kali Carb 200	Useful for backache labours or a posterior presentation. For chilliness after a contraction.	Label as **backache**
Kali Phos 200	For exhaustion or low energy	Label as **exhaustion**
Pulsatilla 200	For weepiness, clinginess, pleading for help. Contractions short, weak or stopped entirely.	Label as **weepy**

Further reading:

- The Family Guide to Homœopathy, Dr Andrew Lockie (Hamish Hamilton) *(available from Active Birth Centre shop)*
- Homœopathy for Mother and Baby, Miranda Castro (Macmillan)

The Helios Homoeopathic Kit for Childbirth can be ordered from www.activebirthcentre.com.

For mail order remedies, or further advice, contact: Helios Homœopathic Pharmacy, 97 Camden Rd, Tunbridge Wells, Kent TN1 2QR. Telephone 01892 537254. Website: www.helios.co.uk

Aromatherapy

Certain essential plant oils can be very helpful in labour and will not clash with homœopathy. As essential oils are very powerful, they need to be used very carefully and combined by an expert for use in labour.

Ready combined aromatherapy oils for massage in labour can be obtained from the ABC by mail order. These can be used in the weeks leading up to labour, as well as during labour itself.

Excellent workshops on the use of aromatherapy massage in pregnancy and labour are offered regularly at the Active Birth Centre.

The essential oils listed below can be used generally for labour. You can use them for massage by mixing five or six drops in a little base oil such as almond oil. Alternatively they can be diluted with a few drops of water and used on an essential oil burner. They can also be added to a cold water spray or used to make an aromatherapy compress. To do this, use a bowl of hand hot water and add 5-6 drops of essential oil. Immerse a towelling face cloth in the water and then wring out and pass to the labouring mother.

You will probably find basic aromatherapy essential oils at your local health food shop or chemist. Special combined oils made up by a skilled aromatherapist are available by mail order from the ABC.

For individual consultations and massage workshops contact the Active Birth Centre.

Further reading:
- Aromatherapy for pregnancy and childbirth, Margaret Fawcett (Element Books)
- Aromatherapy and massage for mother and baby, Allison England (Vermillion)
- Aromatherapy for women and children, Jane Dye (Daniel)

ESSENTIAL OILS FOR USE IN LABOUR

Lavender	Relaxing and soothing. Many women find this oil very helpful for pain relief, or to reduce nausea, to boost energy or to calm emotions.
Marjoram	Relieves muscle pains such as backache. Also calms the mind and helps to change the energy in labour.
Clary Sage	A uterine tonic and relaxant. This will encourage labour and stimulate contractions. Useful when contractions are weak or labour stops. Warming, relaxing, reduces panic. DO NOT USE IN PREGNANCY.

These organic essential oils can be ordered from www.activebirthcentre.com

Transcutaneous Electronic Nerve Stimulation (TENS)

With this method of pain relief, four small adhesive electrode pads are attached to your back on either side of your spine. You control the delivery of low level electrical impulses by using a push button hand-held unit. These travel along your spinal cord to the brain where they compete with pain impulses arising from the uterus, and help to block them. TENS may also stimulate the release of endorphins and raise endorphin levels if used continuously from early labour. Starting early is necessary as it has a cumulative effect.

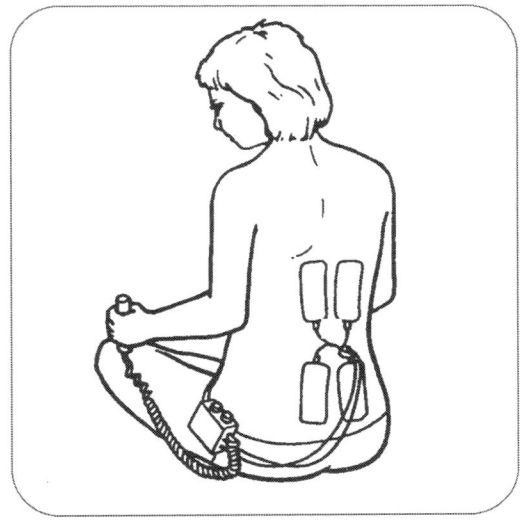

It is important to position the pads correctly and helpful to practise using the unit prior to labour. The machine is adjustable to offer high, medium or low doses of stimulation. It is left on all the time in labour and turned up during contractions.

How effective is TENS?

Feedback from women and findings from various studies are mixed. Some women find TENS very helpful while others do not. Women like the fact that it is self-controlled and harmless. TENS is most useful in the early stages of labour and can be used while travelling to hospital or birth centre in the car.

TENS cannot be used during electronic monitoring of your baby's heartbeat or in water, or on skin which is broken or irritated. It takes half an hour before the endorphin level builds up so the effect will not be felt immediately.

Potential benefits

- Can be used from the very beginning of labour
- Suitable for use at home, while travelling, or in a birth centre or hospital
- No adverse effects on mother or baby.
- Does not affect consciousness or awareness
- Mobility and position changes are possible
- Compatible with other forms of pain relief except back massage, water or electro-acupuncture
- Self administered and can be discontinued easily

TENS machines are available for hire from Birth Tens at www.birthtens.co.uk. Tel: 01455 233808

Maternity Reflexology

Maternity Reflexology is an ancient natural therapy working with the subtle energies in the feet to balance and harmonise the woman's being in pregnancy and after birth. It involves specific massage strokes and pressure, sensitively applied with the hands and thumbs to the feet according to the mirror reflection of all body anatomy and systems, which are reflected in the microcosm of the feet. It is non-invasive and respectful. Experiencing this kind of reflexology throughout pregnancy sets the stage beautifully for an active birth and a deep and pleasant bonding and parenting.

In particular, the reflexology 'priming of labour', for prevention and treatment of overdue labours, is most popular, especially if 2 or 3 reflexology treatments have been received prior to the expected due date. It encourages the timely onset of labour, preparing the mother hormonally and emotionally as well as being a potent work-out. It is also possible to encourage breech babies to turn, after 36 weeks, via specific reflexology techniques.

However the most vital and unique contribution maternity reflexology is able to make is the hormonal balancing treatment. This harmonises all endocrine functions in a very effective way, in particular the hypothalamus- pituitary- adrenal axis which is involved in the secretion of the birth hormones.

The lymphatic drainage routine is also very popular for swollen ankles and feet and general wellbeing.

Maternity reflexology complements active birth yoga beautifully and specifically addresses many of the discomforts of pregnancy and the imbalances of the over adrenalised modern life. Thus a healthier physiological state is fostered during the whole of pregnancy setting the scene for a more wholesome birth and parenting.

Acupuncture

Acupuncture in pregnancy is a safe procedure which can benefit both mother and unborn child. It has many applications and is particularly effective for treating the common complaints of pregnancy. It has within it specifically designed treatments to assist your pregnancy throughout every step from fertilisation to postnatal care, with treatments directed to building up your strength and overall health.

Chinese medicine has been used for thousands of years, combining acupuncture, herbs, nutrition, massage and exercise into one integrated system. One of its main branches is Acupuncture, which aims at restoring the body to a state of balance. Acupuncture achieves this regulation by using very fine needles to stimulate specific areas of the body. These areas are known as acupuncture points and are situated along pathways known as meridians, which bind and unite the body together.

Medical Pain Relief

Your body produces hormones called endorphines during labour which act as natural pain killers. Focusing on the rhythm of your breathing, making sounds, changing positions and moving your body, massage, complementary therapies, immersion in warm water, and TENS are ways to reduce or relieve pain. Sometimes, however, the pain may become intolerable, especially when the labour is prolonged. It is important to recognise when some form of medication is required, and wise to keep an open mind about accepting help if you need it.

All drugs used to relieve pain can have some adverse effects for mother and baby. Some are still inadequately researched, especially in the long-term or subtle effects. All pain-killing drugs cross the placenta and enter the baby's blood stream in the same concentrations as in the mother's blood. To use pain relief most effectively, these adverse effects need to be understood and weighed up against the need for pain relief. Timing and dosage are also very important. Always discuss the methods of medical pain relief on offer with your birth attendants in advance prior to the birth.

In this section the potential benefits and proven risks of each method are listed and then some guidelines are given in summary to help you to make the best use of your obstetric backup. Bear in mind when reading this section that when there is normal progress and you are managing the pain well yourself, the risks of using medical pain relief probably outweigh the benefits. However, if you feel exhausted or the pain is extreme, then the benefits of accepting some pain relief will probably outweigh the risks. Moderate use at the right time, in the appropriate circumstances, can minimise the potential for adverse effects for you or your baby.

It is essential that the extent of cervical dilation be checked by vaginal examination immediately before taking any drug in labour. If full dilation is imminent (7-10cms), it may be better to avoid certain types of pain relief that could affect progress of the second stage or the baby's condition at birth.

Pethidine and meptazinol (may be called Meptid)

These analgesic drugs are powerful narcotics derived from morphine. They act on the nerve cells in the brain and spinal cord to alter your perception of pain. The pain impulses are present but the sensations may be modified. They are given as an intra-muscular injection into the thigh or buttocks.

Effects on the mother

Potential benefits:

- Modification of pain. The majority of women find that pethidine offers ineffectual pain relief, although some do find it helpful.
- Can lower blood pressure and this may be beneficial when the mother has raised blood pressure.
- A low dose can have a relaxant effect, which may help to improve cervical dilation in cases of very slow or ineffectual dilation due to anxiety and tension in reaction to the pain.
- May be a preferable choice for mothers who do not want to use an epidural anaesthetic or inhalation analgesia (gas and air).
- Can be used at a home birth.

Potential risks:

- The amount of pethidine you take (the dosage), as well as the time you take it, will affect the potential adverse effects. Higher or repeated doses will increase the risks (see below for guidelines).
- As well as altering pain perception, pethidine alters consciousness. Some women do find it helpful in coping with pain, but many feel that they lose control, courage, and confidence and do not experience effective pain relief.

- Nausea is a common side effect, so pethidine is often given in combination with Promazine, a powerful tranquilliser used to quell the nausea. Promazine can cause drowsiness and prevent you from giving birth actively, increasing the likelihood of your needing other interventions. Pethidine may be taken without tranquillisers and an anti-emetic drug such as Metoclopramine (which may be called Maxolon), does not cause drowsiness and may be used, if needed.

- In very high or frequently repeated doses, Pethidine may depress the mother's breathing and artificial ventilation may be needed. This slowing down of the mother's breathing lowers the amount of oxygen and increases the levels of carbon dioxide in her blood. This in turn affects the oxygen supply to the baby and may be a cause of foetal distress.

- Pethidine can lower blood pressure which may result in faintness, dizziness or nausea.

- Drowsiness may interfere with your active participation in the birth and psychological interaction with your partner and family.

- May increase the risk of postnatal depression.

- May slow down the progress of labour and diminish your active control of pain as well as the quality and significance of the birth experience.

Effects on the baby:

These drugs do cross the placenta and can have an adverse effect on the baby, the most dangerous of which is foetal distress in labour and the possible depression of the baby's breathing at birth. This is why some babies whose mothers have used large doses of pethidine need to be resuscitated (given oxygen) at birth or may need to be given an antidote drug called Naloxone. The effect on the baby is greater if the baby is small or premature, if the mother receives high doses of pethidine and if these are given near to the time of birth.

In early labour the mother's system helps to remove the pethidine from the baby's blood via the placental circulation, whereas later the drug is more likely to remain in the baby's bloodstream after the birth and take longer to clear.[1] The baby's system will then have the added burden of detoxification, while learning to adapt to life outside the womb. This can lead to the baby being drowsy or sluggish, therefore having sucking difficulties after birth, which can disturb the start of breastfeeding and cause weight loss. In premature babies it can take days before the drug is excreted, increasing the need for support systems to help them breathe and feed. For many such reasons paediatricians generally prefer women to use other forms of pain relief.

Narcotic drugs do affect consciousness and we cannot know how they make the baby feel in the uterus. There is also significant evidence of a correlation between drug addiction in young adults and the use of narcotics in labour.[2]

Guidelines for using pethidine or meptazinol

Dosage and timing are crucial factors in the successful use of pethidine. The dose usually varies depending on the woman's weight, and may be repeated after four hours. The maximum dose usually recommended in hospitals is 150-200mg, and 100-150mg for every repeat dose. However, due to the possible adverse effects on both mother and baby, it is now thought best to use very low doses, with a maximum dose of 50mg. Pethidine is generally best taken neat in a low dose without the addition of a tranquiliser, and before 7cm cervical dilation.

Summary

- Discuss the use of pethidine/meptazinol with your birth partner and midwives prior to the birth.

- Always have an internal examination to check dilation prior to using pethidine. It is generally advisable to avoid using pethidine after 7cm dilation.

- Take a low dose which does not exceed 50mg.

- Avoid combination with tranquillisers - request neat pethidine. If you feel nauseous, request an anti-emetic such as Metoclopromide (Maxolon), which will not cause drowsiness.

- Avoid taking several repeat doses. Consider another method if pain relief is inadequate.

---

1 Gamsu, H., Chambolain, G., Wright, A., Steer, P. Eds. *Pain and it's relief in childbirth.* Edinburgh, Churchill Livingstone, 1993, pp 93-100.
2 Jacobson, B., Nyberg, K. *Opiate addiction in adult offspring through possible imprinting after obstetric treatment.* BMJ 1990, 301:1087-90.

Gas and air (Entonox)

This combination of 50% nitrous oxide and 50% oxygen (laughing gas) is the most common form of anaesthesia used in UK hospitals. It is inhaled through a rubber mask or mouthpiece which you hold yourself. This has a valve that opens when you inhale and closes when you exhale. You should begin to inhale just as you anticipate the start of a contraction. The anaesthetic effect builds up and lasts for 60 seconds, taking the edge off the pain without completely eradicating it. Each breath of gas and air may leave you feeling a little 'high'. Once the contraction reaches its peak, or if you have had enough, you can put the mask down and the effects soon wear off.

Gas and air is best used late in the first stage, during transition. It is only useful for a relatively short time because the anaesthetic effect wears off. Used throughout labour, gas and air can make a woman feel very disconnected from her labour and dependent on the entonox, and it may alter her normal state of consciousness in an unpleasant way. Prolonged use is also very dehydrating. At home births the midwives carry one or two cannisters only, each of which may last for about 30 minutes.

Many women do find a little gas and air very helpful for the final very strong contractions approaching full dilation, but it can sometimes cause confusion and delay the onset of the expulsive reflex in the second stage. However, as the effect is of limited duration, if you do not like it, you can stop using it and the effects will soon wear off.

There is scant research information about the effects of nitrous oxide on the labouring woman and her baby. There has been research which highlights concern about the risks of overexposure to midwives therefore moderate use is now recommended.

Potential benefits

- Gas and air is self-administered so you can have total control of when and how much you take.
- Minimal use with good timing can be effective for temporary pain relief.
- Entonox does not appear to inhibit uterine activity.
- Can be used at home, birth centre or in hospital, and in an ambulance.
- There are fewer clinical side effects than for pethidine and these are not noticeable when used moderately.

Potential risks

- Extensive use throughout first stage may result in loss of power and control, or active participation in pain management.
- The "high" may leave you feeling confused, dizzy or out of control.
- If pain is very intense, the pain relief from Entonox may be inadequate.
- Can cause nausea and vomiting.
- May affect the hormonal changes during transition and delay the onset of the expulsive reflex.
- The mother may focus on inhaling the gas and air in second stage rather than on pushing, and this may slow down the second stage or cause feelings of confusion. It is generally best to avoid the use of Entonox in second stage or to use it very minimally.
- The immediate effect on the baby appears less significant than with pethedine but is still under researched. We do not know how Entonox makes the baby feel or if there are long term effects. One Swedish study has linked teenage amphetamine addiction to long exposure to the gas during birth. [3]

Summary

- Discuss with your birth partner and midwives prior to the birth.
- Try to avoid using Entonox throughout the first stage. Check dilation if necessary.
- Use in late first stage and transition only.
- Use minimally. Start inhaling at the first sign of the contraction beginning. Take two or three inhalations and then put down.

---

[3] Jacobson, B., Nyberg, K., Ekland. G., et al (1988) *Obstetric pain medication and eventual adult amphetamine addiction in offspring.* Acta Obstetrica et Gynecologica. Scandinavia 67-677-82

Epidural anaesthesia

Great advances have been made in epidural technology in recent years and different types of epidural are now available. For this reason it is important to discuss this option with your hospital prior to the birth and to find out what sort of epidural they offer.

The standard epidural

This is a local or regional anaesthetic derived from cocaine (called Bupivicaine) which is injected by a skilled anaesthetist into the lower spine to block the nerve fibres that transmit pain sensations from the uterus. In the first stage of labour, pain from uterine contractions may be prevented by a high block, which should not completely numb your legs. In the second stage, when the pain is felt in the vagina, a lower block may be given. In many hospitals a 'low dose' epidural is offered which uses a minimal dose of anaesthetic, enabling the mother to be aware of contractions without feeling pain.

The mobile epidural

The so-called mobile epidurals represent the latest advance in epidural technology. Whereas a standard epidural tends to numb the pelvic area and the legs, the mobile epidural numbs the pelvic area only. Theoretically this kind of epidural enables mothers to be mobile: to stand, walk, and change positions. However, in practice, most mothers do not feel like moving around very much and although they can use their legs, may not feel very sure where they are! Nevertheless, the use of supported upright positions, such as kneeling over a bean bag, or sitting on a chair leaning forward, are possible and help to encourage the baby's descent, improve circulation to the placenta and reduce some of the risks to mother and baby.

Mobile epidurals are available in many hospitals. This form of anaesthesia is usually inserted lower in the spine. A narcotic drug such as morphine or a combination of narcotic drugs and Bupivicaine are used. When narcotics only are used, their effectiveness tends to wear off in late first stage and a top up Bupivicaine is given. Timing of this is important to prevent 'breakthrough pain'. The onset of pain relief is more rapid than with the standard epidural and there is less shivering.

While some of the risks associated with standard epidurals may be reduced by using a mobile epidural, nausea is more common, and itchy skin is another common side-effect (a drug such as Benedryl, which also causes drowsiness, may be given to combat itching). Women with oral herpes need to be aware that the use of narcotics can stimulate an outbreak and may mean that you will need to avoid kissing your baby.

It is important to discuss the use of low dose or 'mobile' epidurals with your attendants as innovations and research in this technology are progressive and new information may be available after the publication of this booklet.

Spinal anaesthesia

This is similar to an epidural but is quicker and easier to insert. This form of anaesthesia is short-acting and no top-ups are given, so it tends to be used in late labour only, or in second stage for instrumental deliveries and caesarean section. It involves the use of a finer needle as no catheter is inserted. The quality of pain block is said to be better than with epidurals and the onset of anaesthesia is more rapid.

The side effects are similar to those seen with epidurals, only the incidence of headaches is lower with the type of needle used for this procedure. The lower dose of local anaesthetic used for spinals also has a lower risk of toxicity.

A spinal block is injected lower than an epidural, in the base of the spine. It anaesthetises the uterus, vagina and perineum and is often the first choice of pain relief for forceps deliveries.

In summary, spinals can produce rapid and effective anaesthesia for caesarian section while using low doses of local anaesthetic.

EPIDURAL ANAESTHESIA

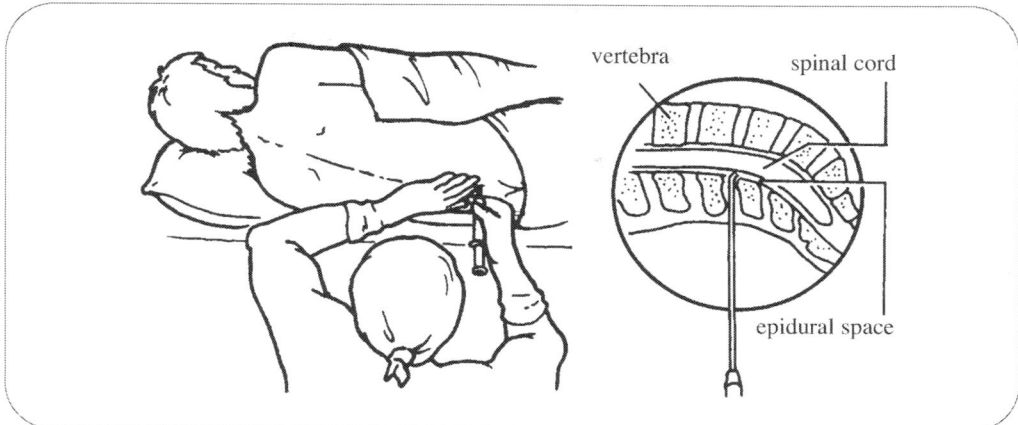

The spinal cord lies within a bony canal which runs through the vertebrae of the spinal column. The vertebrae protect the spinal cord which runs through the centre of the spine. The cord itself is covered by a membrane called the dura, and between this and the vertebral bones is the epidural space.

First an intravenous drip is inserted into the wrist or hand to maintain the mother's fluid levels. Then the woman lies on her side, curled up in a foetal position. If this is uncomfortable, the epidural may be inserted while she is sitting on the edge of the bed leaning forward.

The anaesthetist uses a local anaesthetic to numb the skin and the spinal ligaments and then inserts a needle into the epidural space. A fine cannula, or flexible tube, is threaded down the needle and into the space. The needle is removed and the cannula is taped with elastoplast along the mother's back up to her shoulder where it's end is closed off by means of a sterile filter. Doses of anaesthetic can be topped up painlessly during labour through the filter into the cannula without needing to repeat the insertion.

The anaesthetic effect lasts approximately 1 to 2 hours before a top up is needed. Some hospitals use a top up system and others may use a continuous intravenous drip to administer the epidural anaesthetic. Studies have shown that top ups by midwives are preferable as the amount of anaesthetic used overall is usually less with this system.

Potential benefits of epidural and spinal anaesthesia

- When successful, an epidural is the most effective form of pain relief for childbirth. Studies have shown that pain relief from epidural anaesthesia is satisfactory in 80-85% of cases. It may work only partially with some women and fails for approximately 5% of women.

- An epidural can be very helpful in a prolonged labour if the pain becomes intolerable or if the mother is exhausted, thus enabling her to rest or sleep. In these circumstances a Syntocinon drip (see p31, Induction) may also be used to encourage dilation. Sometimes this break from the pain may enable the mother to recover sufficiently so that she can regain her energy and push her baby out vaginally in second stage. This is often possible if the epidural is designed to wear off at the end of the first stage when the mother is fully dilated.

- An epidural does not affect your mental state so that you remain conscious and alert.

- Epidurals reduce anxiety and fear in some women so that labour may progress better.

- This form of anaesthesia is easy to top up so that minimum doses can be used and consistent pain relief can be maintained.

- Epidurals are useful for a forceps delivery as they eliminate pain and reduce trauma.

- A popular form of anaesthesia for caesarean section, epidurals enable the mother to remain conscious for the birth and enjoy early contact with their baby. They can be used in the next 24 hours for post-operative pain relief and help to encourage a quicker recovery.

- Epidurals lower blood pressure so it may be beneficial for those mothers who have severe pre-eclampsia or a substantial rise in blood pressure.

- Can be useful for a premature labour.

Potential risks

The potential risks of using an epidural for mother and baby are significant. However, careful attention to the dosage and timing and selective use in the appropriate circumstances will minimise the risks. Research into epidurals is considered by many experts to be insufficient to justify its widespread routine use, and often parents are not fully informed about the potential risks. While the list of risks may appear daunting when you read them all at once, bear in mind that careful use can help to prevent these potential effects.

Mother

- Rarely, the anaesthetist may be able to achieve only partial blockage of sensation so that pain or pressure may be felt in one segment of the body, or on one side only.

- Occasionally the needle may penetrate the dura causing leakage of the spinal fluid with severe migraine like headaches after birth. This can disturb early contact with the baby. This can be medically treated with a blood patch.

- The mother's blood pressure may fall as the blood vessels in the lower body dilate causing the blood to pool within them. This can result in queasiness or faintness and the possible use of drugs called vasopressors. This may also reduce placental blood flow and possibly result in less oxygen going to the baby, increasing the potential for foetal distress. Because of this, every woman having an epidural needs to be on an intravenous drip to top up the volume of her blood.

- Injury to the lower spine and pelvic joints can occur during birth as a result of loss of sensation in extreme positions,.so that the woman is unaware of over extension. Care and sensitivity by birth attendants can help to prevent this problem. Some women also complain of backache due to injury after an epidural, and this can be a common long-term problem postnatally.[4]

- Temporary paralysis of the pelvic muscles removes the natural stimulus for the baby's head to turn in the pelvic canal, and reduces the mother's urge to bear down. Because of this, the pushing reflex may be inhibited and a forceps delivery or caesarean section becomes more likely. In some hospitals, up to 20% of epidurals lead to forceps births. One study showed that only 46 out of 100 first time mothers will avoid a caesarean section or ventouse/forceps delivery if they choose an epidural. However, a low dose epidural can be allowed to wear off at the end of the first stage, and the mother can be helped into an upright position. Working with her contractions and gravity will greatly increase her chances of a spontaneous vaginal birth. This approach is becoming a more realistic option with the wider availability of "low dose" and "mobile" epidurals in many hospitals.

- Malpresentations are more likely with epidural as the mother cannot help to position the baby with her instinctive movements as she would do normally, and the pelvic muscles are less effective. This increases the chance of an instrumental delivery or a caesarean section.

- Because a woman on an epidural does not breathe as heavily as she would if she were feeling the contractions, she loses a natural way of cooling her body by exhaling. As a result, some women experience a rise in body temperature and unnecessary treatment with antibiotics, or it may mask a genuine fever.

- The use of an epidural anaesthesia may slow down the progress of labour resulting in the additional use of syntocinon to enhance contractions. This may be avoided by keeping sensory stimulation and disturbances to a minimum to encourage hormone secretion and maintain the contractions.

- Shivering is a common side effect of epidurals.

- While the pain relief gained from an epidural can make birth a positive event, some women may feel that they were deprived of fully experiencing the labour and birth.

---

4. Macarthur, Lewis M, and Knox E.G. *Health after childbirth*. HMSO 1991.

- When the epidural wears off, the nerves are often very sensitive and a caesarean scar or an episiotomy may feel excessively painful for a short time.
- Some women have swollen or painful feet for 4-5 days after the birth.
- If the anaesthetic is accidentally injected into the spinal cord, this may result in paralysis of the respiratory muscles, necessitating artificial ventilation. Epidurals should therefore only be undertaken when ventilation is possible. This is a very rare occurrence.

Baby

Little is known about the long term or subtle effects of epidurals, and there has been remarkably little research in this area. However, there is evidence that the anaesthetic is present in the baby's blood and brain cells after the birth. Some studies now show that epidurals do have an effect on the baby, altering breathing rate and blood sugar levels. Low doses of epidural anaesthetic and good timing will help to reduce the potential risks to the baby, which include:

- Foetal distress. Because of their effect on the mother and her loss of mobility, epidurals increase the risk of foetal distress. It is not uncommon for abnormal heartbeat patterns to occur, resulting in the need for instrumental delivery or caesarean section. The risk of foetal distress can be decreased if the mother lies on her side rather than her back, to reduce pressure on the blood vessels in front of her spine, thus aiding blood circulation to the placenta. Changing sides from time to time, with the midwife's assistance, is a good idea. The back rest should be raised so the mother is lying with her head higher than her pelvis.
- If Syntocinon is used to speed up the labour, the baby will be exposed to the combined effects of this (see Induction p.31) as well as the epidural.
- Sometimes babies who have been exposed to large amounts of Bupivicaine in-utero are born slightly blue in colour. This is due to imperfect oxygenation of the mother's blood and these babies may be unresponsive to their surroundings for a little while after birth until they recover, or need paediatric assistance.
- If the mother has an "epidural fever" this may result in a rise in the baby's temperature too, and may lead to treatment with antibiotics or special care in a separate baby unit after birth.
- The use of epidural has been shown to result in irritability and inconsolable crying in some newborn babies who may be slow to "settle" after birth and need patience and understanding. They may be very sensitive to noise and have some difficulty latching on to the breast at first and inefficient sucking. Treatment of the baby with cranial osteopathy can be very helpful as soon as possible after birth.

Recommendations for the use of epidurals

- Appropriate use, minimum dosage and minimum duration will maximise the benefits and minimise the risks.
- Always ask for an internal vaginal examination to check dilation just before an epidural is inserted. Unless needed for an instrumental delivery, epidurals are usually best avoided after 7cms dilation, or they may affect your ability to push and increase the risk of forceps or caesarean section. You might consider an alternative at this time, such as getting into a water pool or gas and air (entonox).
- If the mobile epidural is available it may be preferable. To minimise the potential risks, this can be used for pain relief if pain becomes unbearable, rather than being used from the outset for a "pain free labour".
- Low dose epidurals are preferable and easy to top up if necessary.
- Intermittent top ups are usually preferable to a continuous drip.
- Lie on your side, well propped up on a bean bag or cushions, and ask your midwife to help you to change sides periodically. It may be possible to kneel over a bean bag or sit on a chair besides the bed leaning forward onto pillows, or to stand leaning forward if a low dose or mobile epidural is used.
- If using a mobile, discuss the possibility of "breakthrough pain" with your midwife so that careful timing of the top up can avoid discomfort.
- Ask for the most senior anaesthetist to insert the epidural. Request that he or she allow the epidural to wear off when you are fully dilated. Wait for the second stage contractions to begin (this may take some

time after an epidural). Your partner or a helper can sit on the edge of the bed or a chair. You can be helped to slowly get off the bed and onto your feet. You can then use your partner for support and squat for the birth. You can use a deep squat position between your partner's knees if you are used to it, or a more upright 'standing squat' or sit on your partner's knees, if that is more comfortable. Allow time for the contractions to become effective. With the help of gravity, many women succeed in giving birth vaginally after an epidural using this approach.

Other forms of medical pain relief

Pudendal block

Pudendal block has been largely superceded by epidural anaesthesia which offers more complete pain relief, but it may be useful for a low forceps delivery or for an episiotomy. A local anaesthetic is given, via a needle inserted through the vaginal wall, to block the pudendal nerve as it emerges from the side of the pelvic outlet. This removes all sensation from the lower third of the vagina and from the skin of the labia and the perineum.

Perineal block

This is the most commonly used anaesthesia apart from gas and air. An injection, effective within three or four minutes, is used to numb the perineum before an episiotomy is carried out, or a tear repaired. The anaesthetic is injected directly into the area to be stitched and may sting as it is inserted. The area is then numb for about 90 minutes, long enough for the repair to be done.

General anaesthesia

A general anaesthetic may be needed for caesarean section, a mid-cavity forceps delivery or removal of a retained placenta. Because it may be needed in an emergency, women are asked to eat small amounts and to drink only sips of water during established labour. This reduces the risk of the stomach contents being inhaled into the lungs. To prevent this, once the mother is unconscious, a tube is passed into the airway via the mouth. Both baby and mother are taken into account when the anaesthetic is given. Sleep is induced with an injection of an appropriate drug, followed by another to induce muscle relaxation which allows the airway tube to be inserted. The mother then inhales further anaesthetic gases to maintain unconsciousness. Once the operation is over, the anaesthetic agents are exhaled by the mother and she slowly recovers consciousness. It may be a while before she is ready to have first contact with her baby. The baby may be sleepy and very occasionally may need to be resuscitated. Usually, however, the first contact and breastfeeding can take place within one hour after the birth. Treatment with homoeopathy soon after the birth can be very helpful in eliminating the toxic effects of the anaesthetic for both mother and baby, and can aid healing and recovery.

An alternative to medical pain relief - using a birth pool

The use of a birth pool during labour and for birth is an option which is increasingly widely available at home, in birth centres and hospitals for 'low risk' mothers. Entering a pool of warm water at around body temperature when you are half way through labour (at around 5-6 cms) is a way to achieve a much deeper level of comfort, support and relaxation just when you need it most. For many women this can provide an alternative route to medical pain relief. Research has shown that when the option of a water birth pool is available, fewer women need epidurals. It is certainly worth trying the pool for half an hour – chances are that you will forget all about needing pain relief – or you can still

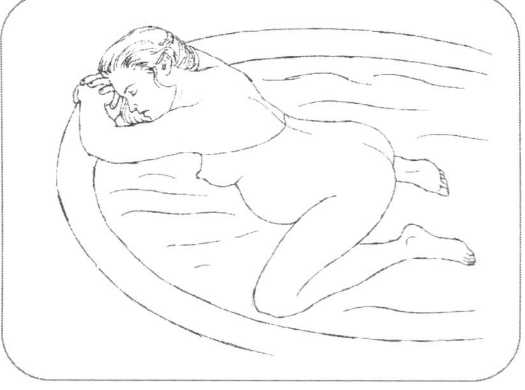

get out and decide to have an epidural. Using a birth pool in active labour may increase the possibility of a natural, intervention free birth. Studies have shown that women rate this option very highly. A waterproof hand held sonic aid monitor is used to check the baby's heart rate while you are in the pool.

The main benefits of using a birth pool in labour are:

- Due to a short-term increase in the secretion of oxytocin, contractions may be more effective and yet less painful.
- You may find that you can move and change positions much more easily.
- You will feel a greater sense of privacy.
- Because your body weight is supported in the water, you can rest more easily during and in-between contractions.
- The duration of your labour may be shorter and before long you may be ready to give birth.

Birth in water

It may also be appropriate for the baby to be born in water in the pool. This generally happens when progress in the second stage is good and the mother does not want to leave the pool. Being born in water is a lovely, gentle and calm way for a baby to be welcomed to the world and may also be more comfortable and easier for the mother. During the birth, while still under water, babies often open their eyes, unfurl their limbs and move towards the surface. The baby is lifted out of the water within 10 seconds of the birth and the first breath is stimulated as the face makes contact with the atmosphere. Up until then the 'dive reflex' suppresses breathing and the baby still gets oxygenated blood through the cord. If you are planning a water birth, you do need to be ready to change the agenda if it doesn't seem the best way for your baby to be born at the time. If contractions seem to be slowing and losing their power in water, oxytocin levels may be falling and you may need to get back to gravity outside the pool to stimulate and strengthen contractions for the birth and the delivery of the placenta.

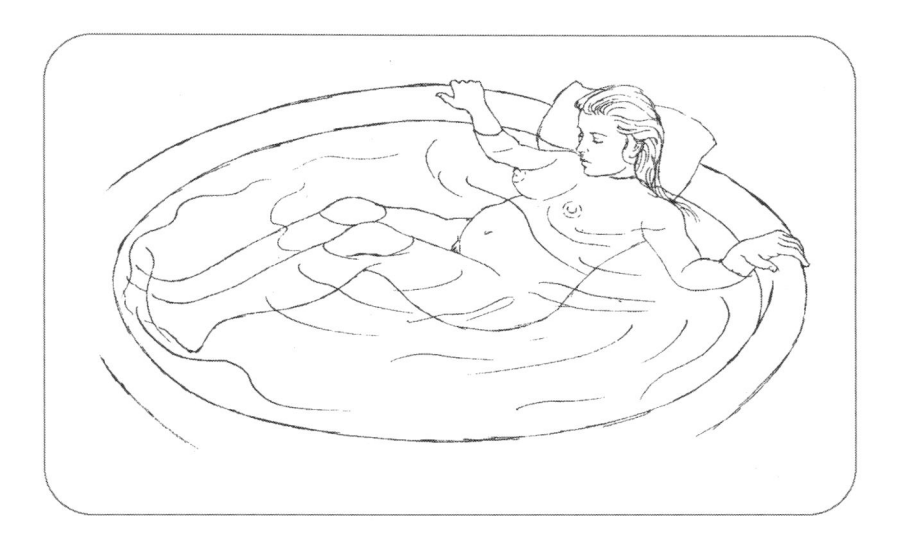

Recommended reading:
- The Water Birth book by Janet Balaskas
- Water and Birth DVD

Both available from www.activebirthcentre.com

Guidelines for reducing and relieving pain in labour

Non-medical methods:

- Change the environment to one which is more 'hormone-enhancing' by increasing privacy, darkening the room etc.

- Try a change of position, or different movements and focus on 'grounding' with the exhalations through the parts of your body which are in contact with the floor.

- Use a concentrated focus on your breathing, positive visualisation and release sounds freely. Breathe away the pain when you exhale.

- Try some massage using aromatherapy oils for pain relief, or diffuse the appropriate oils in the room on an essential oil burner.

- Use warm water - a birth pool, bath or shower

- Use homœopathic remedies such as Arnica, beginning in early labour.

- Use TENS beginning in early labour.

- Acupuncture, acupressure, reflexology and self-hypnosis may all be helpful in increasing your ability to cope with pain.

- Have a trusted birth partner with you throughout labour

Medical methods:

- Always have an internal examination to assess dilation before opting for medical pain relief.

- Before 7-8 cms dilation you could consider either an epidural or a low dose of pethidine if dilation is slow. It is best to avoid repeated doses of pethidine.

- Epidural top-ups can be timed so that the anaesthetic will wear off just as you are ready to push the baby out.

- After 7-8 cms dilation, try minimal use of gas and air.

Induction

The word menstruation comes from the old English 'mona' which means moon. Since time immemorial women all over the world have calculated the length of pregnancy as some time during the tenth cycle of the moon after the last menstruation.

Women of the Chagga tribe of Uganda would mark the months of pregnancy by making notches on pieces of bark.

Amongst the Manus of New Guinea, little bundles of sticks are kept as moon counters. When ten bundles have been collected, the mother knows that her baby is ready to be born.[1]

In Malaysia, traditional midwives expect labour to begin when the woman's feet and ankles become cold, indicating that the body heat is moving towards the womb.[2]

Jacqueline Vincent Priya, in her book 'Birth Traditions and Modern Pregnancy Care' says:

"When I talked to pregnant women from traditional societies, their happy vagueness about when the birth was likely to take place always amused me. After my own experiences with modern doctors who provided a specific 'B-day' and started to worry if the baby hadn't arrived by that date, the relaxed attitude of these women was a tonic. They usually knew within a month or so as to when the baby might arrive and trusted their own internal knowledge and experience of the pregnancy as to when the birth would take place."

She goes on to describe some of the special rituals used traditionally to ensure that the mother goes into labour relaxed and confident.[3] This seems a very long way indeed from the experiences of pregnant women approaching birth in our culture.

In the UK the length of pregnancy is normally calculated as 40 weeks after the first day of the mother's last menstrual period. Estimates of the baby's due date are often made using an ultrasound scan which are not generally accurate to the day.

The vast majority of women begin labour spontaneously when their babies are mature and ready to be born. When labour is initiated before it begins spontaneously, this is known as 'induction.' Routine induction has been described as the 'most predictable way of creating abnormal labour and the need for operative delivery.'

Premature and postmature babies

While these terms are often used without justification, a baby may be genuinely premature or postmature. A premature baby is at risk because the lungs may not yet be ready to breathe air independently, while the main danger to a postmature baby is that the placenta may no longer work well enough to provide sufficient oxygen to the baby. This is called 'placental insufficiency'. Both these conditions are potentially dangerous to the baby and do need medical attention and supervision.

Valid reasons for an induction

- **Placental insufficiency** — if the baby is not receiving enough nourishment through the placenta, induction is often suggested, although the procedure requires careful monitoring since the baby is at risk and the induction itself can be hazardous (see below). Many people believe that a caesarian section may be a safer option.

---

1. Dunham C., and others. *Mamatoto* Virago Press, 1991.
2. Jackson D. *Eve's Wisdom.* Duncan Baird, 1999.
3. Vincent Priya J. *Birth Traditions and Modern Pregnancy Care.* Element, 1992.

- **Multiple pregnancy** — induction may be necessary if one child is receiving less nourishment than the other(s). If you are overdue with twins and induction is being recommended, it may be wisest to accept.
- **Diabetes** — improved methods of diabetes control mean that even severely insulin-dependent women can often go into labour spontaneously at term.
- **Congenital abnormality** — very rarely an induction is done because the baby is abnormal or has died.
- **High risk mothers** — induction is more common in a number of well-defined high-risk groups such as malnourished women, smokers and women with high blood pressure.

Questionable reasons for an induction

- **Disproportion** — occasionally an induction is proposed before the expected delivery date because a previous baby was thought to be too large for the mother's pelvis. The risks of induction may outweigh any potential benefit.
- **Breech presentation** — this is not a valid reason for induction.
- **'Small for dates' baby** — on its own this is not an indicator for induction unless there is also a significant risk of placental insufficiency.
- **Postmaturity** — even if birth has not occurred within a week or two of the expected delivery date, induction is probably unnecessary if mother and baby show no signs of any problems. Induction should only be done in cases where tests indicate placental insufficiency.
- **Convenience** — induction of labour for the convenience of birth attendants cannot be justified, and induction for the convenience of the parents should be carefully considered in the light of the possible risks to the baby.

What to do when you're overdue!

The following information has been produced to help you to be aware of some of the issues that may arise when pregnancy continues beyond the estimated due date, and to empower you for wise decision making.

Your EDD (estimated due date) has probably been in your mind since your first ante-natal checkup. It can be very disappointing and frustrating to find that you are still pregnant a week or more beyond this date. Added to the normal discomforts of the final weeks of pregnancy, you may well feel very fed up and desperate for labour to start, especially when people around you keep phoning to find out if you have had the baby yet, and the hospital is talking about booking a date to induce labour. This can be a very vulnerable time. However you may not be genuinely 'overdue' at all, and unless there is a medical problem, you can take your time to assess the situation and consider the options.

Induction of labour is a contentious subject, yet many hospitals have a policy of routinely inducing after a certain date. Sometimes induction of labour is strongly recommended between 41-42 weeks as this has been shown by research to reduce the overall (very small) number of babies who die in childbirth in the UK (approximately 4-5 babies out of 1000 are likely to die just before or soon after birth and an even smaller number in labour).[4] It has been estimated that when induction is done routinely, approximately 500 women are induced before 42 weeks to potentially save one baby. However this does not mean that induction is appropriate or safe for everyone, nor does it address the other potential hazards, risks and consequences of routine induction policies.

Marjory Tew, the renowned statistician, says in her book *'Safer Childbirth?'*:

'Confirmation is hard to find that induction reduces the danger of perinatal death even in the medical complications for which it is advocated'. [5]

---

4. Anderson T. *Post-term Pregnancy.* The Practising Midwife, Dec 1999. Vol 2, no 11, pp 10–12.
5. Tew, M. *Safer childbirth?* Chapman and Hall, 1995, pp 263.

It has also been shown that convenience is another non medical factor underlying induction policies. Since the advent of induction, studies have shown birth to be more common on weekdays.[6]

There are many doctors and midwives who are critical of routine induction policies and who prefer to follow a different approach. This involves assessing each woman who is 'overdue' individually and then deciding what would be best for her and her baby. The aim is to determine whether the pregnancy is normal (albeit longer than the estimated average length), or whether there are any signs of post maturity such as slowing of the baby's heart rate or a very low amniotic fluid level and therefore cause for concern or possible intervention.

Genuine post maturity can endanger the baby, so a thorough assessment will provide the information needed when deciding whether to induce or not. [7] An induction would only be performed if the risk of the baby remaining in the uterus was considered greater than those associated with inducing. Sometimes, if the baby is thought to be at great risk, a caesarean section may be the preferable option.

The decision making process should involve the parents and take their views into account. Legally they are not obliged to agree to an induction, whether or not it is hospital policy. However if there are convincing signs of post maturity, if there is an existing medical or health problem or if you are having twins, where the risks of prolonged pregnancy are greater, it is best to follow the advice of your midwife or obstetrician. Other reasons to induce may include progressive high blood pressure or pre- eclampsia, convincing indications of placental insufficiency and slow growth of the baby, significantly reduced amniotic fluid which is outside of the normal range, premature rupture of membranes with an extended period of no contractions (beyond 48 hours), or failure to progress in labour (this is called augmentation or acceleration of a labour which has already started).

Before deciding whether or not to induce labour, the following can be considered:

- Estimated due date. The length of a normal pregnancy may be anywhere between 37-43 weeks and, very rarely, can even extend beyond this. If conception occurred later than the average estimate of day 14 of the menstrual cycle (i.e. with an irregular or longer menstrual cycle) this may be the reason that the baby is not yet ready for birth and labour hasn't started. Ultrasound scan estimates of the due date are approximate and are not always accurate. The usual method of estimating the average length of normal labour (nine months and one week since the first day of the last menstrual period) is known as Naegele's rule and was first established in the mid 19th century. There has been no satisfactory evaluation of this method and it has been shown that the results from obstetric 'wheels' made by different manufacturers used to calculate the length of pregnancy are not consistent [8]. Research has shown that the average length of pregnancy may be 41 weeks and one day for many women with a 28 day cycle. Japanese and black women tend to have shorter pregnancies than white Americans. There is a wide range of variation in the length of a normal pregnancy. [9]

- There is also a lot of controversy about the normal length of human gestation and therefore over the definition of post-term pregnancy. The normal length of gestation for babies is variable. Babies initiate labour themselves when their lungs are ready for breathing, by releasing hormones into the amniotic fluid. These are absorbed into the mothers bloodstream and act as messengers to her brain. This kicks off the release of the hormone oxytocin which gets contractions going and starts labour. Being born too early may mean that maturation of the baby's lungs is not yet complete. That is why premature babies often need help to start breathing. If labour is induced when the dates are wrong, the baby may be born prematurely and have problems breathing, possibly needing special care.

- Mother and baby's well being. If routine checks reveal no sign of anything abnormal in either mother or baby, then there is no pressing reason to intervene by inducing labour. Another option is to reassess the situation on a daily basis and to continue waiting for nature to take its course, provided there are no

---

6. Macfarlane, A. *Variations In Numbers Of Births And Perinatal Mortality By Day Of The Week In England And Wales.* British Medical Journal, Vol. 2, 1978, pp 1670–73.
7. Chamberlain, C and Zander, L. *Induction.* British Medical Journal, Vol. 318, April 1999, pp 995–998.
8. McParland, P and Johnson, H. *Time to Reinvent the Wheel.* British Journal of Obstetrics and Gynaecology, 1993, Vol 100, pp 1061–1062
9. Hutchon, DJR. *Expert Analysis Of Menstrual And Ultrasound Data In Pregnancy – Gestational Dating.* Journal of Obstetrics and Gynaecology, Vol 18, no 5, Sept 1998, pp 435–438.

problems. After 42 weeks, daily monitoring of the baby's heartbeat is recommended. This may necessitate a daily visit to the hospital and is the most reliable way to check the baby's well being. A consistently satisfactory heartbeat indicates that the baby is getting enough oxygen and the placenta is functioning normally.

- An ultrasound scan. This may help to assess the size of the baby, the volume of amniotic fluid, the placental function and to provide more information about the baby's well being. If clinical monitoring and an ultrasound scan confirm normal development of the baby then the pregnancy can continue.

- A second opinion. Since there are known risks attached to medical induction, seeking a second obstetric opinion is justified unless the need to induce is urgent. Try to find an obstetrician who does not have a strictly interventionist approach. This can include an ultrasound scan.

- Take note of any encouraging signs that labour is imminent. These may include more frequent or mild contractions which may stop and start, a mucous discharge or 'show', unusual back pain, or feeling a bit 'spaced out'. Your midwife may tell you that the cervix has softened, moved forward or has dilated to 1 or 2 cms. You may experience diarrhoea as the bowel starts to empty or there may be some leaking of the amniotic fluid or the membranes may break. Also, don't worry if none of these are happening - not everyone experiences these changes prior to the onset of labour. Try to be patient, relax and take it easy without being unduly stressed or anxious. If there are no problems, then everything is on course and you will go into labour when your baby is ready. This is a great time to indulge in a pampering treat like a wonderful aromatherapy massage.

> If you do decide to opt for an induction, you can consider the natural methods first unless the need to induce is urgent. All methods of induction, natural or medical, are likely to work best when carried out as close as possible to the day when your baby is ready to be born and labour is imminent.

Natural methods of inducing labour

The following suggestions may help to initiate labour:

- Get some gentle exercise such as walking, swimming or doing yoga. Meditate and relax every day to stay in tune with your baby and your inner guidance.

- Acupuncture and/or reflexology combined with homœopathy can be very effective in helping to get labour started. It's best to consult a specialised practitioner with experience in this area. Alternatively, most complementary therapies can help to initiate labour, especially if you have already been having treatment during your pregnancy.

- Wait as long as possible and then try a glass or two (no more!) of good organic wine one evening.

- Provided your membranes haven't broken, you could try making love. There are natural prostaglandins in semen which soften the cervix, and nipple stimulation may also help to release more oxytocin, the hormone that makes the uterus contract.

- Your midwife could do a 'cervical sweep' - a massage around the cervical opening. This may stimulate the secretion of natural prostaglandins which soften and 'ripen' the cervix and help to start labour. This may be uncomfortable but has been shown by research to be effective. You should always be consulted and agree to this procedure beforehand. [10]

- Drink three cups of organic raspberry leaf tea per day. This is a mild uterine tonic and stimulant.

---

10. Boulvain, M and others. *Does Sweeping Of The Membranes Reduce The Need For Formal Induction Of Labour?* Journal of Obstetrics and Gynaecology, Vol 105, no 1, Jan 1998, pp 34–40.

- Evening primrose oil is said to be helpful in ripening the cervix. You can take three capsules of 500mg every day from 36 weeks until birth.

Medical methods of induction

Prostaglandin gel or pessaries (Prostin)

The discovery of synthetic prostaglandin, similar to that found in the lower segment of the uterus, represented a major breakthrough for induction.

If medical induction is the selected option, it is generally recommended to try prostaglandin first, as this is the least invasive method of induction. This method is preferable to a drip as it leaves the mother free to walk about, and it does not necessarily involve breaking the waters.

It should be possible to use a birth pool or to proceed with an active birth after successful induction with prostaglandin.

Prostaglandin is applied by a midwife or doctor using a small applicator into the vagina. This may help to soften and ripen the cervix and trigger labour. This needs to be done in hospital as mother and baby's reactions are unpredictable. Contractions may begin very soon or up to four applications at 6 hourly intervals may be necessary. Low doses of 1mg of Prostaglandin (maximum of 4mg in 24 hours) will help to prevent this occurrence. Occasionally with first time mothers if the cervix is still very unripe, the first dose may be 2mg.

If Prostaglandin induction is successful, labour can proceed as it would normally. If it does not result in contractions, then the next step is to break the waters and then progress to induce with a Syntocinon drip if this is not successful. Some doctors will agree to wait another day or so and try again, but this is not usually the case. If these methods are both unsuccessful, a caesarian section will be done. Hence, it is unwise to embark on the use of prostaglandin unless there is a very good reason for induction in the first place.

Because of the risk of over-stimulating the uterus, prostaglandin should not be given to a woman whose cervix is already partly dilated. Some women react very rapidly to prostaglandin so its power should not be underestimated. Prostaglandin can only be administered in a hospital as a strong reaction in the mother may also affect the baby.

Very rarely, extremely intense and painful contractions can occur and this can deprive the baby of oxygen and result in foetal distress.

Prostaglandin can occasionally irritate the smooth muscle of the bowel, causing vomiting, diarrhoea or migraine, and the pessaries may cause vaginal irritation.

New drugs are being developed which may soften the cervix more effectively than prostaglandin. However extreme caution and adequate research is needed before introducing these for widespread use, so make sure you know what drug is being applied.

Syntocinon drip

This powerful stimulant of uterine activity is a synthetic oxytocic drug designed to imitate the oxytocin produced by the pituitary glands of both mother and baby. It can be used to accelerate or augment a labour that is proceeding slowly, as well as for induction. While Syntocinon stimulates uterine contractions effectively, it will inhibit the secretion of natural oxytocin and does not have the 'bonding' effect of the 'love hormone'.

It is usually given by means of an intravenous drip. This generally restricts the woman's movement, although mobile drips are available. The drip will be kept in throughout labour to ensure that contractions continue, until well after birth. Syntocinon usually begins to work almost immediately.

Induction of labour can be carefully designed to mimic what would happen in a normal labour and when well managed, is often successful. However there are a number of potential risks to be considered which include the following:

- Induction often makes labour progress more quickly and intensely. This is because the artificial hormone

Syntocinon is fed intravenously into the mother's bloodstream in much higher concentrations than the gradually increasing level of hormones her body would produce naturally. This means that contractions may be longer and stronger and harder to cope with. Days of pre-labour uterine activity may be condensed into a few hours.

- The overall recovery time between contractions, (when fresh oxygenated blood reaches the placenta) may be shorter. Therefore the risk is that, over time, the baby receives less oxygen than would otherwise be the case. This may be demanding on the baby and increases the potential for foetal distress and, therefore, the likelihood of a caesarean section. Frequent or continuous monitoring of the baby's heartbeat to check how well the baby is coping is essential when labour is induced.

- The strength of the contractions will also be monitored continuously to detect any signs of overstimulation. When the uterus is overstimulated uterine activity becomes uncoordinated and the cervix may fail to dilate. In extreme cases the uterine muscle may go into spasm, resulting in foetal distress.

- Postpartum haemorrhage is more likely because an overstimulated uterus is less responsive to natural oxytocin or the similar synthetic drugs which can be used in the third stage of labour to deliver the placenta and membranes. Syntometrine should therefore always be used in the third stage following an induction with Syntocinon.

- The pain with an induction may be greater from the start and, with no natural build-up, there may be no time for the mother to adjust. The contractions can also have two peaks. More intense contractions also result in more pain, so the likelihood of needing an epidural is greater, as is the risk of the baby being delivered eventually by forceps, ventouse or caesarean section.

- In large doses, Syntocinon may cause oedema and high blood pressure.

- While some inductions are successful, this is not always the case. Approximately 10-30% of inductions fail and in this case the baby needs to be born by caesarean section. [11]

Possible complications for the baby

- There is a chance that the baby may be born prematurely, especially if dates are wrong. Induction should only be done if the risks of continuing the pregnancy are thought to be greater than the risks of prematurity. Breathing difficulties are more common when labour is induced, especially if the baby is premature and has immature lungs.

- Foetal Distress - the increased strength and duration of contractions in an induced labour can reduce blood flow to the placenta, possibly resulting in distress and a delivery by caesarian. Very rarely, severe oxygen deprivation can result in brain damage but this eventuality can be prevented by careful monitoring.

- Syntocinon has also been linked with an increased risk of neonatal jaundice.

What you can do to avoid complications

Many of the potential problems may be avoided with careful management. The following suggestions may help:

- By using comfortable upright positions such as kneeling on the bed over a beanbag, sitting on a chair leaning forward onto the bed, or lying well propped up on one side, you can ensure a better blood supply to the uterus than there would be if you lie on your back or semi-recline. In upright positions there is no direct pressure from the weight of the baby on the large blood vessels which supply the uterus as there is when reclining. This allows for better circulation to and from the placenta and helps to minimise the risk of foetal distress.

- Being upright may also help you to cope better with the contractions. In second stage supported upright positions, which engage the help of gravity, will help you to push more effectively.

- As contractions may be intense almost right away, bear in mind that it will take about half an hour before

---

11. Enkin, M., et al. 1991. *Effective Care In Pregnancy And Childbirth* (1st Edition; Oxford University Press.

your natural pain killers or endorphins 'catch up'. It is helpful and reassuring to have someone with you at all times and to focus on breathing over the peak of the contractions. (Try long slow releasing out breaths through the mouth which 'take away the pain', with relaxed in breaths through the nose). Some women do manage without medical pain relief this way, however you can (and should!) have an epidural if the pain is unmanageable.

- You can also request that the drip is introduced as slowly as possible and you can ask for the drip to be slowed down if you find it overwhelming.
- Careful use of the minimum dose of syntocinon needed to be effective, combined with supported upright positioning, will help to prevent overstimulation of the uterus and foetal distress.

ARM - Artificial rupture of membranes .

This procedure – also known as amniotomy and "breaking the waters" is no longer recommended as a method of starting labour. ARM is carried out by inserting a plastic instrument resembling a crochet hook through the cervix to puncture the membranes. This is invasive and may be uncomfortable or painful. ARM can also be used as a way of accelerating a slow labour that has already started. Although sometimes done unnecessarily, this may be a good idea if the mother is becoming exhausted and ordinary patience and other less invasive methods don't work (see accelerating labour, below). It may also be helpful late in labour, if there is a long delay, to stimulate the onset of the second stage.

If ARM is suggested to induce labour, ask for an explanation of the reasons why it is being recommended. Its use as a way of inducing labour has some serious potential side effects and can profoundly alter the course of labour. It is, however, still often routinely done in conjunction with the use of Prostaglandin or Syntocinon. You may request not to have the membranes ruptured as a matter of course when being induced.

Potential problems when inducing labour with ARM

- Rupturing the membranes often stimulates the immediate onset of very intense contractions which the mother may find difficult, or too intense and painful to cope with, as they come on suddenly without the gradual build-up of a natural labour. The level of endorphins her body produces does not yet match a sudden increase in the intensity of contractions so other forms of pain relief may be necessary, with their attendant risks.
- It also increases the risk of an ascending infection by removing the protective barrier of the membranes. If there is an infection, then a caesarian section will usually be done.
- The outcome of ARM is unpredictable. If labour is not established within a reasonable time, further interventions are likely to be recommended. A caesarian section may be suggested if the baby is not born within 24 hours.
- ARM alters the intra-uterine pressure and removes the protective cushion of forewaters around the baby's head. This can cause compression of the umbilical vessels and trauma to the baby's head during the second stage.

Accelerating labour

Each labour has its own rhythm. It is perfectly normal for labour to slow down or to stop for a while and usually, with patience and faith, contractions will start again and become stronger. If labour slows down or stops, try to rest in a darkened room or to sleep. You may also need to eat and drink. Provided the midwife is satisfied that your baby and yourself are showing no abnormal signs, then there is no harm in waiting. The baby's heart beat should be checked from time to time while you are resting. If your labour is going very slowly or not progressing well and you are exhausted, it is important to alternate periods of rest with periods where you can try the following ideas:

- Darken the room and ask all but essential helpers to leave the room, or try to be alone for a while. Increasing privacy may help to boost your hormone secretion.
- Squatting often intensifies contractions. Use a stool to avoid fatigue, and squat during or between contractions.
- Walking, moving or changing to a more upright position may help.
- Express any feelings or fears you may be holding on to – have a good cry if necessary. Holding back emotions can hold back labour.
- Entering a water pool can be an effective way to stimulate weak contractions. If not available, try a bath or shower. Sometimes in a long labour contractions slow down in a birth pool but this is an interval in which the mother can rest and relax and regain energy.
- Nipple stimulation by massage may stimulate more efficient uterine contractions.
- Try Caulophyllum (see Homeopathy p.14) or Clary Sage (see Aromatherapy p.15). There are many ways that complementary therapies can help to make contractions more effective. Seek expert advice if you are in contact with a practitioner.
- If all else fails, then ARM, Epidural and/or Syntocinon drip may be used to help you reach full dilation. When these methods are used appropriately as a last resort, the side effects are usually minimal and the outcome successful. You can relax and accept the help you need and enjoy your birth knowing you have done your best.
- Occasionally, Syntocinon may be used to stimulate contractions in the second stage when the urge to push does not occur after a long wait, or the mother is exhausted and contractions are weak.

At the end of the day

Birth is unpredictable and doesn't always go according to our plans or expectations.

If you manage to avoid a routine induction, the efforts you made to assess the situation may feel very worthwhile in retrospect. On the other hand, if the wisest decision at the time was to opt for an induction, you may feel really pleased with the way things went. Or you could feel disappointed that labour didn't start spontaneously, particularly if this necessitated other interventions being used or a caesarean section. When labour is induced and actively managed, control passes from the mother to her attendants. If she feels that the induction was unnecessary, she may feel angry, resentful and violated. It is also natural, after an induction, to wonder what a spontaneous labour might have been like and whether you made the right decisions.

It is important to talk through your feelings afterwards, either way. Every birth has its ups and downs and this process of 'debriefing' after the event is always helpful . Once you have done this, try to let go of the 'what ifs' and 'might have beens', accept what happened as what was meant to be, then put the experience behind you and move on. As new parents you have plenty to do and a newborn baby to enjoy. When labour is induced for good reasons, there is no need to feel that you have failed in any way.

Producing a live and healthy baby is an enormous achievement, so try not to let your experience of birth become more important than your baby, and remember to appreciate yourself for doing so well!

Guidelines for medical induction

- Request a thorough assessment and explanation of the situation and procedures, which may include seeking a second opinion on the necessity of induction in your case, and an ultrasound scan. In the absence of a medical problem, you may decide to wait as long as possible before inducing with natural or medical methods. In this case daily monitoring and reassessment of the situation is recommended after 42 weeks.

- Try natural methods first, unless induction is urgent.

- If you have decided to be medically induced you could first try Prostaglandin, as this is the least invasive procedure. If it works, labour may progress normally. If a Syntocinon drip is used the application of prostaglandin first helps to prevent overstimulation of the uterus.

- Request the minimum effective dose of either Prostaglandin or Syntocinon.

- Request a mobile drip with a long lead if available. Ask to have it sited in the forearm of the hand you use least, in order to limit your mobility as little as possible. If possible, arrange yourself comfortably over a beanbag and pillows, in a kneeling position leaning forward so that your trunk is supported and you can rest completely between contractions. The arm with the drip attached can be supported by pillows. Kneeling will help you to deal with the intensity of the contractions, reduce pain and improve circulation to the baby, and so reduce the risk of foetal distress. It may also be possible to sit on a chair beside the bed and lean forward on to cushions.

- Expect the first contractions to be difficult to cope with. Their intensity may ease within 30 minutes when your natural endorphin levels will have had a chance to increase to match the power and frequency of the contractions. Try to wait 30 minutess or so before deciding whether or not to have an epidural.

- Ask for the drip to be phased in very slowly and gently and focus on 'breathing away' the pain with long exhalations through the mouth and relaxed inhalations. Focusing on your breathing, especially the exhalations, during contractions, can be very helpful and enables many women to cope with an induced birth without painkillers.

- Monitoring can be done just as easily in the kneeling or sitting position as when you are semi-reclining, using frequent sonicaid, a belt monitor or a scalp electrode (if the baby is distressed or at risk). Some women find the belt monitors uncomfortable, some find continuous monitoring very reassuring when attached to a drip.

- The speed of a Syntocinon drip can be regulated so if you are finding the contractions too fast and intense you can ask the midwife to turn it down.

- It can be very frightening being alone, strapped to a monitor and attached to various forms of equipment during an induction. Emotional support is crucial. Ask the midwife, student midwife or nurse to stay with you at all times other than to pop out briefly. This will ensure that any problem is quickly noticed.

The third stage controversy

A physiological third stage

When labour and birth progress normally, the third stage can usually also continue without any intervention. This is called a 'physiological third stage' and unfolds in the following way:

The baby is born, usually with the mother upright. Privacy is paramount throughout the third stage until the placenta is delivered and it is also important for the room to be very warm, even overheated. This is to encourage optimal hormone secretion and good strong uterine contractions and to facilitate the first contact between mother and baby.

The baby is placed, for a few minutes, on an absorbent towel on the floor between the mother's legs on his or her belly in the safety position, or may be passed to the mother directly. The amniotic fluid in the baby's lungs drains during birth, or is absorbed before breathing begins.

If the baby is born in a birthing pool or bath, he is gently guided to the surface of the water into his mother's arms. He will begin to breathe once his face is out of the water and comes into contact with the air. Some birth attendants will request a woman to come out of the bath or pool for the third stage although this is not considered necessary by others. When leaving the pool it is best if the mother holds the baby as she climbs out of the pool and then sits down on a soft surface beside the pool to continue with the first contact undisturbed.

First contact between mother and baby takes place and the first touching occurs. The mother sits upright so that gravity can assist the separation of the placenta. The umbilical cord is not cut but left to cease pulsating naturally while the baby begins to breathe. Breathing starts as soon as the cooler air of the atmosphere stimulates nerve endings around the baby's nose and mouth. As the baby takes its first breaths and its lungs expand for the first time, it is still receiving oxygen from its mother via the placenta and the pulsating cord.

The mother may have already picked up, or been handed, the baby. If not, she does so now, and the first eye-to-eye and skin-to-skin contact occurs.

During this time, the baby's breathing is established and the cord stops pulsating once the baby no longer needs oxygen from the placenta.

The baby makes contact with the breast and may begin to suckle. Stimulation of the nerve endings in the nipple brings about the release of more oxytocin from the mother's brain. This will stimulate the uterus to contract so that the placenta separates from the lining of the womb.

There is further secretion of hormones which makes the uterus contract, stimulated by the release of emotion, skin-to-skin, and eye-to-eye contact as the baby begins to suck.

Uterine contractions or 'after pains' expel the placenta and membranes.

After the placenta is expelled, the cord can be clamped and cut. Sometimes it is cut earlier, after pulsation has completely ceased.

The uterus continues to contract strongly when the baby sucks. This results in tightening of the blood vessels at the placental site so that bleeding ceases and the uterus begins to retract back into the pelvis. Within an hour of birth it is about the size of a large grapefruit.

In the days that follow, the uterus continues to retract back to normal every time the baby feeds. The lining of the womb (lochia) is gradually shed, rather like a long period which slowly diminishes and stops.

Within 4-6 weeks, the uterus will have returned to its pre-pregnant state.

Routine management of the third stage of labour

There is intense controversy within the medical profession about how to 'manage' the third stage of labour. Many doctors and midwives advocate a physiological third stage for those mothers who have had a normal labour and birth. However, in many places, routine induction of the third stage with syntometrine is common practice.

Syntometrine is a drug which is usually injected into the mother's buttock or thigh as the baby's shoulders are being born or immediately after the birth. It consists of 5 units of syntocinon and 0.5mg of ergometrine. The syntocinon causes the womb to contract strongly within two or three minutes of the injection and the ergometrine causes a further and sustained contraction of the lower uterus and cervix some seven minutes after the injection.

When syntometrine is given, the midwife or doctor will then want to deliver the placenta before the action of the ergometrine, which could trap it inside the uterus. Therefore the cord is clamped immediately before it stops pulsating to prevent the syntometrine getting into the placental circulation and a large rush of placental blood going to the baby when the uterus contracts. Then the placenta is delivered by controlled cord traction (pulling on the cord) soon after the first contraction caused by the syntocinon is felt.

This practice evolved as a response to the problems of postpartum haemorrhage in the days when most women gave birth lying down and then became a routine intervention.

Some possible problems with a routinely managed third stage:

- The placenta could be trapped inside resulting in the need for removal of the placenta under anaesthetic.
- A fragment of placenta may remain inside and may cause an infection necessitating treatment with antibiotics.
- Due to premature clamping of the cord the baby may be undertransfused and therefore miss the benefit of the nutrients in the last blood coming from the placenta. Alternatively the baby could be overtransfused which is considered to be a possible cause of neonatal jaundice.
- Very rarely the uterus may invert due to controlled cord traction.
- The first contact between mother and baby is disturbed and the natural hormonal balance altered.
- The mother may feel severe cramps and nausea for a short time

Benefits of routine management

There is very little evidence to support the implementation of routine induction of the third stage. However, a trial at Hinchingbrook Hospital showed a slightly higher rate of post partum haemorrhage in women who had a physiological third stage compared to those whose third stage was routinely managed [12]. (This study also concluded that there was no evidence to support the hypothesis that upright positions cause significantly more post partum haemorrhage than supine positions in third stage.)

This outcome came as a surprise to advocates of the physiological approach who maintain that further research is needed before routine induction of the third stage can be justified. Michel Odent [13] was critical of the study on two counts: Firstly, the study excluded women with lower haemoglobin levels normally associated with good perinatal outcomes. He also commented that the environment was not fully sensitive to the mother's privacy. He stresses the need for warmth, silence and a total lack of disturbance in the third stage to enhance optimal bonding and hormone secretion to contract the uterus most efficiently and prevent bleeding. Misunderstanding of the paramount importance of privacy is common in the third stage.

---

12. Rogers J, Wood J, McCandlish R, Ayers S, Truesdale A, Elbourne D. *Active versus expectant management of third stage of labour: The Hinchingbrooke randomised controlled trial.* Lancet 1998; 351: 693–699.

13. Odent M. *Active versus expectant management of third stage of labour.* Lancet May 1998; Vol 351 p 1659.

The third stage of an active birth

An active birth is, in itself, a preventative of postpartum haemorrhage. When the mother is upright the physiological processes are assisted by gravity with the least possible stress on the uterus and placenta. If the mother is sitting upright after the birth, the placental separation and retraction of the uterus are made easier and more efficient due to the effect of gravity, and blood does not 'pool' in the uterus but flows out of the body. Blood loss can therefore be accurately assessed and there is less risk of infection. Because of the 'pooling' effect, when a mother lies down in the third stage, some of the normal blood loss stays in the uterus. (N.B. If the midwife is not used to seeing women remaining upright in the physiological third stage, that which is normal blood loss may seem to be more than she is used to seeing.)

The undisturbed first contact between mother and baby and the first breastfeeding stimulate the release of a very high level of the hormone oxytocin which results in very strong contractions to expel the placenta and seal the placental site.

When the mother is undisturbed, the likelihood of postpartum haemorrhage is reduced after an active birth and routine induction with syntometrine is not generally necessary. However, it is wise to have syntometrine easily available so that, on the rare occasion that blood loss after the birth is more than normal, it can be given to those women who need it.

Guidelines for the use of Syntometrine

In the appropriate circumstances, Syntometrine can help to stop excessive bleeding and can therefore be invaluable when used for the right reasons.

- You have the right to refuse routine use of Syntometrine, but would be unwise to do so if you are bleeding more than is usual, or if the delivery was assisted with forceps or ventouse, or you have had your labour induced or accelerated, because these interventions increase the risk of postpartum haemorrhage.

- If you have had a normal physiological labour and birth without drugs or interventions and there is no sign of unusual bleeding, you may wish to ask the midwife not to use Syntometrine.

- If bleeding seems excessive, Syntometrine can be given immediately. Intramuscularly, the drug takes 2-3 minutes to take effect. In an emergency, it can be given intravenously by injection and will act in about 40 seconds but not all midwives are trained to give intravenous injections, so it is advisable to find out if this is possible before you make a decision to refuse it in the first instance.

- Unless the need is urgent, Syntometrine may also be given after the cord has stopped pulsating and been cut, rather than just as the baby is being born. This will help to avoid some of the risks outlined above.

- Sometimes after a home birth, the midwife may wish to give the mother a dose of Syntometrine before she leaves to ensure there is no haemorrhage in the hours following the birth. However, if the baby is sucking well and the uterus has contracted down nicely, this may not be necessary.

- Since the use or non-use of Syntometrine is so controversial, it is important to find out the policy of your birth attendants and discuss the issue long before the birth. Make sure that your wishes are recorded and attached to your notes if you would rather 'wait and see' if you need Syntometrine rather than be given it routinely, or if you would prefer it to be administered after the cord stops pulsating. At all costs, try to avoid a confrontation on this issue while you are actually giving birth.

Assisting Babies to be Born

Episiotomy

When birth is active, an episiotomy is rarely needed. However, it is the simplest way of assisting the baby to be born quickly if there are difficulties, or in an emergency.

An episiotomy is a surgical incision beginning on the back wall of the vagina and extending into the skin of the vagina and perineum and the underlying muscles. There are two types of episiotomy— midline and medio-lateral. The midline cuts directly backward from the vagina, stopping short of the anus. The medio-lateral starts off like the midline, but then goes out to one side to avoid the anus. The midline cut is usually preferable because it runs between muscles, not through them, and is done as far as possible away from large blood vessels and nerves. It is also less painful while healing. Occasionally during birth the midline cut may extend into the anus but a skilled midwife can prevent this kind of 'third degree' tear.

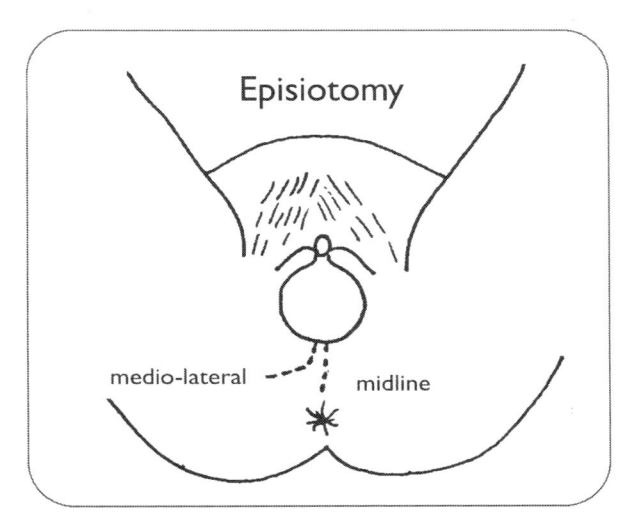

Episiotomy used to be done routinely in some hospitals for all first births allegedly to 'protect' the perineum and prevent tears. However, they are now less common.

A tear is a natural hazard of birth. Most tears are minor, involving only the superficial layers of the vagina and the labia. They heal easily and are known as 'first degree' tears. Occasionally more severe 'second degree' tears occur involving the underlying muscles. Tears generally heal better and are less painful than episiotomies. The uneven line of the tear may be more difficult to stitch but the subsequent ease of healing makes up for this. Minor tears may not need stitching at all. With the use of upright postures during childbirth, episiotomy is rarely necessary.

How to avoid tearing and episiotomy

- Preparing in advance

    Pregnancy yoga and breathing will help to improve circulation to the perineum and enable you to learn how to relax and release these tissues with the breath when you are giving birth.

    Perineal massage in the last month of pregnancy may help to increase the stretchability of the tissues.

- Help in labour

    The birth should not be hurried, while the midwife guides you to release the baby slowly, allowing the tissues time to relax. Spontaneous ejection of the baby will reduce the possibility of a tear.

- Gravity effective postures

    The most effective way of avoiding a tear is to give birth in an upright position and to wait for the natural expulsive reflex to occur, thus avoiding strenuous pushing. If you are lying on your back the pressure of the baby's head is directed down on to the perineum and the muscles between the vagina and the anus are subjected to maximum tension. In vertical positions the pressure is brought forward and spread evenly throughout the vagina so that the perineum can release spontaneously as the baby's head emerges.

    In the supported squatting positions, tears tend to be superficial, around the skin of the vaginal outlet instead of at the muscular back wall of the vagina. They are easily stitched if necessary, and do not cause much postnatal discomfort or pain. Second degree tears are rare, third degree even rarer. First degree tears may heal naturally and not require stitching.

- If the baby is slow to emerge, supporting the perineum with warm compresses will bring blood to the tissues, helping them to expand and stretch. This is also very soothing. After the birth of the baby's head, gentle delivery of the shoulders prevents tearing.
- Labouring in water may soften the perineal tissues allowing them to expand more easily and thus prevent tearing or the need for episiotomy.

Perineal Massage

The perineum involves the skin and muscles in the area between the vagina and the anus. This massage, done during the last month of pregnancy, helps to prepare this area for the stretching needed for birth - hopefully without tears or need for an episiotomy.

The massage is best done by a caring person, usually the woman's partner, and does a lot to develop the co-operation, use of feedback and touch that you will need during labour. Many women prefer to do the massage themselves, with the aid of a propped-up mirror.

You will need:

- a small amount of unscented massage oil *
- a clock to time the massage
- plenty of pillows

Pick a time of day when you are both relaxed and free from interruptions. The massager will first need to clip the fingernails of the index and middle fingers and wash hands well. The mother can settle into a semi-reclining position that she can really relax in, with pillows supporting her lower back, neck, head and each thigh. If pillows are positioned under each knee, she will not have to use her leg muscles to hold her knees out of the way. Also, she should not pull her knees/thighs too close to her upper body - this puts too much tension on the perineum.

When the mother is relaxed and ready, the partner should dip two fingers in the oil and slowly and gently insert them only about one inch into the entrance of the vagina. First, feel if the perineal muscles are relaxed. The mother should breathe deeply, relax and consciously 'let go' of these muscles. If it is hard to tell if you are relaxing, first tighten with a pelvic floor exercise then let go and relax them. A lot of feedback is helpful here. The massager should be sure that there isn't contact with the higher muscles of the vagina, which the mother has less control over, so don't go deeper than one inch.

The massage itself involves a slow, gentle pulling down and out of the perineum. Be sure that you are using plenty of oil to avoid uncomfortable friction on the skin. Stay in the lower third of the vaginal opening and pull the skin gently down and out (as the baby's head will do). You should feel a slight burning sensation, but not pain. If you can't eliminate discomfort by going slower, pulling less or using more oil, discontinue the massage for the day and try again tomorrow. If you are tense and 'endure it' the stretching will not work. You must be relaxed.

If you are doing the massage yourself, you may find it easier to half kneel with one leg up and place the mirror on the floor underneath you, working into the perineal tissues with your thumb. Then change legs and do the same on the other side.

...

* You can get an organic unscented oil blended especially for perineal massage from www.activebirthcentre.com

Perineal Massage ...

Timing:

- up to 2 minutes for the first 2 weeks
- up to 5 minutes for the second 2 weeks

Discontinue if the waters break or leak, if labour starts, or if you go much past your due date. Most people report a noticeable change in the consistency and stretchability of the perineum after only a week or more of starting this daily massage.

Benefits of this massage include stretching and increasing the elasticity of the perineum and vaginal opening as well as teaching the mother to actively relax her perineum when there is a sensation of pressure on it.

How episiotomy is done

Episiotomies were traditionally performed with the woman reclining. A local anaesthetic is injected to numb the area and the cut is done during a contraction. At a water birth an episiotomy can be performed under water, but this is very rarely necessary.

When episiotomy is necessary

If the vaginal outlet is tight, an episiotomy may be needed. It may also be required if forceps are needed to deliver the baby. The size of the episiotomy can be kept to a minimum by removing the forceps when the head crowns so that the mother can give birth by her own efforts. Vacuum extractors or ventouse fit directly onto the top of the baby's head and do not stretch the vagina as much as forceps.

There is some disagreement as to whether an episiotomy should be routine in a premature birth to protect the baby's head. Although almost always unnecessary, if there is any delay and the head is under pressure, an episiotomy is done.

One argument often used in favour of episiotomy is that it prevents excessive stretching and reduces the risk of vaginal prolapse in later life. Vaginal prolapse has become much less common in the last forty years or so but there is no evidence to suggest that episiotomy is the reason for that. The best prevention of prolapse is to regularly practise pelvic floor exercises during and after pregnancy.

Repairing tears and episiotomies

An episiotomy or tear is stitched by the doctor or midwife, often with the mother lying on her back with her legs in stirrups. Her head and neck should be comfortably supported by pillows and she may like to hold the baby.

Stitching is tedious but should not be painful if a local anaesthetic is given. The best time to be stitched is after you have had a chance to hold your baby, but before the area feels tender. First the local anaesthetic is injected into the area to be stitched. This may be painful but quickly numbs the area. Breathe as you did during contractions and have gas and air to hand should you want it. Once the perineum is numb, the vaginal skin, the torn muscle and finally the external skin are stitched. Usually dissolving thread is used and the stitches do not need to be removed.

The immediate postnatal period

Discomfort and some pain are usual in the first day or two and pain can be severe, especially with a large medio-lateral episiotomy. Pain-relieving tablets and pessaries or even an injection may be needed. These should be kept to a minimum however, as the drug will cross into the breastmilk. Grazes or tears on the front of the labia may cause burning on passing urine but this can be helped by pouring warm water from a large jug over the area at the same time, or sitting in a large bowl of warm water on the toilet seat as you urinate. The burning will cease as the tissues heal.

Sitting on a rubber ring or child's swimming ring will reduce the pressure on the area. Homœopathic hypercal or calendula tincture (not cream), applied locally, will promote healing. Add 20 drops to a little previously boiled water. If you have piles, perhaps brought about by the efforts of labour, these may increase the pain. Women are often afraid of opening their bowels after childbirth for fear that the stitches may burst. This never happens but you may feel happier if you lubricate the anus with olive oil or a haemorrhoid cream.

A large episiotomy sometimes causes muscle spasm and urine retention.

Healing and care of the genital area after the birth

Immediately after childbirth you should wash and bathe the vaginal area twice a day and keep the perineum dry since wetness delays healing. Pat dry gently with a clean towel after each wash. Doing pelvic floor exercises will encourage blood flow and healing. Use of a soothing and antiseptic healing herbal bath is highly recommended for tears and episiotomies (*available by mail order from www.activebirthcentre.com*). Applying concentrated Vitamin E oil to the area every day after bathing during the stage when the scar feels itchy will strengthen the tissues and promote healing.

At first, wait until healing is complete before making love. Gentle penetration is sensible and is easier if your partner is only half erect. The outer area is usually the most tender, particularly at the back of the vaginal entrance. First lubricate the whole area thoroughly with a lubricant or pure oil. Initially, avoid lying flat on your back with your partner on top as this position puts the most pressure on the stitch line. More comfortable alternatives are for the woman to be on top, or for the couple to lie side by side.

Postnatal complications

Pain from stitches will normally disappear within ten days after the birth. Any pain that goes on for longer needs to be investigated. A common reason is a local reaction to the stitches, causing tenderness, particularly at the vaginal entrance, which resolves with time.

Infection along the stitchline is a rare complication, more likely after a medio-lateral episiotomy because swollen, bruised muscles encourage bacteria. It is treated with antibiotics. Alternatively, a herbal compress can be made with slippery elm, golden seal and comfrey root (1 tsp. of each rolled in gauze and steeped in boiling water) can be applied while still warm three times daily.

Very occasionally the wound opens up. It usually heals by itself but the cut may need to be thoroughly cleaned and then restitched.

Deep pain often arises from the lower spine and sacrum, which may have twisted during the birth. The sacrum then pulls the underlying muscles and ligaments that attach to it, so creating tension and pain at the episiotomy site. This may also make intercourse painful. This pain may be relieved by cranial osteopathy or gentle yoga exercises for the lower spine.

If the birth was difficult, painful stitches may be the focus of psychological pain and anger. Many women feel especially violated if they believe that an episiotomy was unnecessary. Sometimes these feelings may not surface at the time, because of the joy of having a new baby, but they can emerge months or even years later.

Very rarely indeed, stitching makes the vaginal outlet too tight for penetration during sexual intercourse, and restitching is needed. Usually, however, when couples think they have this problem, enlightened counselling is the real solution. Women may feel invaded by the birth to such an extent that they can no longer relax their vaginal muscles to allow penetration, so great is their need to hold themselves in and regain privacy. A man may have found it upsetting to watch an episiotomy or to see his partner being stitched. This can alter his sexual behaviour for months. He may be afraid of injuring his partner. The best way to prevent this is to have your partner stand beside you and support you emotionally or hold your hand without watching the procedure.

Ventouse (vacuum extraction) or forceps

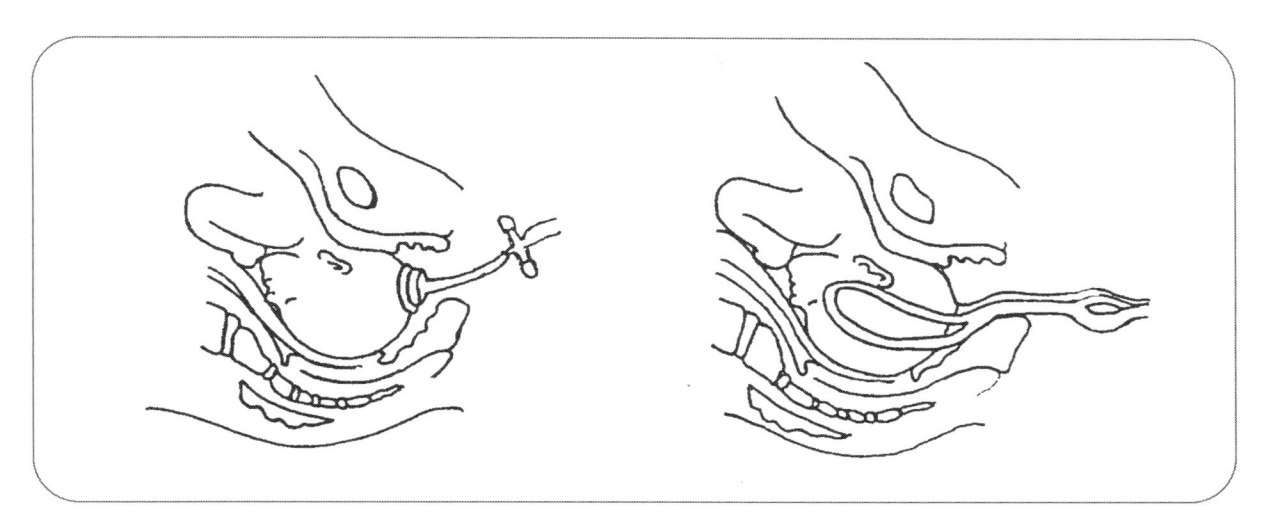

Babies can be assisted to be born with the help of a ventouse or vacuum extraction. This is a rubber cup connected to a vacuum pump which is applied through the mother's vagina to the baby's scalp. A vacuum is created so that the cup remains attached to the scalp by suction, upon which the pull is applied.

Alternatively, forceps may be used. These consist of two metal instruments shaped like large salad spoons with a hole in the middle. They are inserted through the vagina with the help of an episiotomy and applied to each side of the baby's head, and traction is applied to adjust the position of the baby's head and then help the baby out.

Forceps are still used in Great Britain but ventouse is now more widely available. In most European countries forceps have been replaced by ventouse. Safety is thought to be comparable. Although not always the case, some discomfort or trauma may be caused to the baby with both methods. Vacuum extraction is more comfortable and less invasive for the mother and may not require the use of episiotomy or anaesthesia.

If you would prefer to use ventouse should the need arise, discuss this beforehand with your attendants and find out if this method is available.

When an assisted delivery is really justified, it can save the baby's life and prevent unnecessary damage or trauma. When this is the case, it is usually acceptable to the mother and a good outcome with a good recovery follows. Vacuum extraction or forceps are used in about 20% of births and many of these cases of intervention could be prevented by the use of gravity-effective positions in the second stage of labour.

The involuntary expulsive reflex (spontaneous urge to push) of the second stage is easily disturbed and this can be prevented by maintaining privacy and minimising distractions for the mother during transition from labour (first stage) into birth (second stage). Widespread use of epidurals is a common cause of the high statistics for intervective birth.

What you can do to avoid an assisted birth

- Good nourishment and adequate physical preparation in pregnancy.

- Avoid epidural anaesthesia if it is not necessary, or using upright positions in second stage after an epidural.

- Empty the bladder frequently during labour and before the second stage.

- Use upright, gravity-effective positions in labour and second stage to reduce the risk of foetal distress, position the baby well and make the baby's descent through the pelvis as easy as possible.

  In the event of a slow or difficult second stage try positions such as a 'hanging' squat with your arms around your partner's shoulders, or a standing squat leaning forward onto the end of the bed, which may help to bring the baby's head down. A supported standing squat is the most vertical and therefore the more gravity effective position for birth.

- Wait to begin pushing until you feel the urge to bear down, then breathe instinctively through the contractions. You may need to discuss this in advance with your medical attendants.

- Avoid hospitals which have high levels of caesarean, forceps and ventouse deliveries.

When an assisted delivery is necessary

If the baby's head is difficult to deliver, the second stage may be prolonged. If the head is large in relation to the mother's pelvis, or if the baby is in the OP (occipito posterior) position, contractions often slow down and an assisted delivery may be necessary. Ventouse or forceps are used to correct the abnormal position and to provide the additional force needed to deliver the baby. If the baby is breech, forceps are sometimes used to ease the birth of the head, especially if an epidural has also been given. An active breech birth does not usually require forceps, although it may require an episiotomy.

Assisted delivery is more common when epidural anaesthesia has been used because this slows down contractions, removes the natural urge to bear down and push, and relaxes the pelvic floor muscles so that the baby's head is not encouraged to rotate in the second stage.

If the baby suffers severe foetal distress in the second stage of labour, ventouse or forceps can be life-saving by achieving rapid delivery. These interventions are occasionally used to protect the mother. Women who have severe high blood pressure, lung or heart disease may be advised not to bear down and an assisted delivery may be more appropriate.

Conditions for a ventouse or forceps delivery

- The cervix must be fully dilated and the bladder empty.
- The head must be engaged in the mother's pelvis (if the head is still high a caesarian may be necessary).
- Sometimes delivery must be assisted when the baby's head is low down in the birth canal, but the mother is too anaesthetised or tired to push her out. This is known as a 'lift out' delivery, needing only a local anaesthetic to numb the birth outlet.
- Occasionally, if the baby is lodged a little further up the pelvic cavity (particularly in cases of OP presentation) ventouse or forceps extraction are used in what is known as a 'mid-cavity' delivery. This would usually require an epidural or spinal anaesthetic. The other common reason for a mid-cavity delivery is when an epidural has affected the mother's urge to bear down.

What happens during an assisted delivery

The mother is asked to lie on her back with her legs supported by stirrups. You can ask that your partner stay with you throughout, although its not necessary or recommended for your partner to observe the procedure. Your partner could to sit next to you at the top of the delivery table while a screen blocks off the view of the delivery.

In a ventouse delivery the cup is inserted into the vagina and fitted on to the baby's scalp. It takes a few minutes for suction to build up between the cup and the baby's head and then traction is applied during a contraction to help the head to descend. An episiotomy is not always needed because the suction cap does not take up any space along the sides of the vagina, unlike forceps.

In a forceps delivery, local anaesthetic is injected into the perineal area before the episiotomy is done. Then the blades are inserted into the vagina to cradle either side of the baby's head. Holding them together at the handle, the obstetrician applies traction during two or three contractions to help the baby out. In between the contractions, the pressure is relieved.

If the baby is in occipito posterior (OP) position, an assisted delivery may involve rotation of the baby's head to the anterior position. This can be done manually by the obstetrician, or with a vacuum cup or specially shaped forceps. After rotation, the mother's own bearing down efforts may be enough to deliver the baby, with minimal help from the obstetrician.

What an assisted delivery is like for the baby

In a vacuum delivery, the baby may feel the suction on her scalp and the pull through the head and neck. The pulling force is exerted for a minute at a time. Sometimes the baby is born wihout any sign of an assisted delivery, but she may be born with a round, swollen, red area on the crown of her head which will take a few days to subside.

During a forceps delivery, the baby will feel the instruments along the side of her head and the pulling force of the forceps during two or three contractions, for a minute at a time, and may experience a strong tug in her head and neck. She may be born with marks on the cheeks and ears, which will usually disappear within a few days.

A skilled obstetrician, aware of the possible effects on the baby, will sensitively apply the minimum force to assist the birth. Most babies make a rapid recovery after an assisted birth but, because they may have a sore head and feel irritable, they may need to be handled very gently during the first few days. This usually subsides quickly, especially with the help of plenty of close body contact.

You can help to reduce trauma and bruising to yourself and your baby by taking the homœopathic remedy Arnica 200 just before the birth, and then keep taking it three times daily until bruising is gone. The baby can be given a dose of Arnica 6 as well, but discuss this first with a homœopath. A visit to the cranial osteopath following an instrumental delivery, in the first days or weeks after the birth, will help to heal the baby of any after effects, and will be equally good for you.

How you may feel

Women often feel sore and bruised, especially after a forceps delivery. Episiotomy, stitches and pelvic pain are more common with these procedures.

If you know that your baby might not have been safely delivered without help you will probably feel relief and gratitude. If the ventouse or forceps were skillfully used, you may not have had much pain or too great a sense of invasion. If, however, you feel some disappointment at not having achieved a natural birth its wise to acknowledge these feelings, accepting that you are entitled to be disappointed if you wanted something that did not happen.

Your emotions will need to be understood and resolved after the birth. You could begin by talking to the midwife who takes care of you postnatally, as well as the doctor who performed the procedure. Usually these feelings can be resolved in a few weeks but if they continue or are a source of postnatal depression or stress, you should consider expert counselling, otherwise your enjoyment of your baby's first few months may be affected.

Repeat ventouse or forceps deliveries

Ventouse or forceps are most commonly used for a first baby, subsequent deliveries usually being quicker and easier, even if the baby is larger. If you are keen to avoid a second assisted delivery, follow the suggestions above and discuss your thoughts with your midwives during pregnancy.

If ventouse or forceps were used because your first baby was in occipito posterior position, subsequent babies may not be. Even if the next one is OP, your cervix will probably dilate and the pelvic tissues open more readily, and the second stage may be easier.

If the reason for assisted delivery was the size or shape of your pelvis, a repeat assisted birth or a caesarian section may be needed. However, each baby is an individual and the next baby may have a smaller head or be in a better position.

Caesarean section

When the caesarian section operation is performed, the baby is delivered through surgical incisions made in the mother's abdomen and uterus. Then the placenta and the membranes are delivered and the incisions are closed with stitches. The modern caesarean section has become much safer and can be a life saving intervention. Today, new techniques used for caesarian sections enable minimal use of surgical incisions and have led to the expression 'the safe caesarian'.

Why a caesarian may be needed

Caesarian sections are performed either for the health of the mother or, more often, the safety of the baby. Possible reasons include a baby thought to be too large to come through the mother's pelvis; a baby in an untenable position for a normal delivery; a baby suffering from foetal distress, a prolonged labour, or a failed induction of labour.

Maternal reasons for caesarians are less common. The mother's life may be in danger, perhaps from severe pre-eclampsia. There may be severe bleeding, perhaps caused by placenta praevia or placental abruption. The mother may be having an active outbreak of genital herpes, although this is does not always necessitate a caesarean section.

While unnecessary caesarians can be avoided, it is reassuring that modern skill and expertise generally ensure a positive outcome for mother and baby if a caesarian does prove to be essential.

Types of caesarean

It may be that, when you discuss the future birth of your child with your doctor and midwife, you all agree that a caesarian is the most appropriate option in the circumstances, and a date is set for you to be admitted to hospital before labour begins. This is known as an elective caesarian. In contrast, a caesarian may be carried out as an emergency procedure once labour has begun. Modern obstetric units are equipped to deal with such an emergency at any time.

Caesarians also differ in terms of which form of anaesthesia is used. Until 20 years ago, all caesarians were performed under a general anaesthetic, which meant that the mother was unconscious throughout the birth and could not see her baby until she recovered, some time afterward. Today, epidural or spinal anaesthesia provides an alternative which allows you to remain conscious throughout the operation. Postnatal recovery is usually quicker and an epidural is usually safer for the baby.

An epidural caesarian cannot be commenced as quickly, so a general anaesthetic is always used in a true emergency. Some women find the prospect of being conscious during the operation unappealing and prefer a general anaesthetic.

Hospitals vary in allowing partners to be present. Most encourage this during epidural caesareans but usually do not if a general anaesthetic is needed.

The operation

Due to modern anaesthesia a caesarian section is usually a painless procedure. Before a caesarian section your abdomen is shaved and prepared for surgery. After anaesthesia is administered, a catheter (a narrow tube) is inserted into the urethra to the bladder to drain urine, and an intravenous drip is inserted into your arm. The skin of the abdomen is disinfected and the surgeon cuts through the tissues to reach the membranes of the amniotic sac and the baby.

The skin incision is usually a horizontal 'bikini line' cut along the pubic hair line across the bottom of the abdomen. This has the advantage of running along natural lines in the tissues which means less bleeding, less pain and faster healing. In some emergencies, a vertical skin cut is still occasionally used, which runs from below the navel to the hair line. A little less awkward for the obstetrician, it results in a more disfiguring scar. The incision in the uterus itself is usually horizontal and made in its lower segment (called a lower segment caesarian). This reduces bleeding and minimises the risk of scar rupture in a subsequent labour.

The baby is then lifted out, occasionally with the help of forceps. The time that elapses from the incision to the birth is about five minutes. The umbilical cord is clamped and cut, and the baby is handed to the assistant. If you are having an epidural caesarian, you will then be given the baby to hold or, if he is present, the father could take her. Sometimes the paediatrician present needs to examine the baby quickly before passing her to your partner.

The placenta is delivered and checked and then the layers of the uterus and abdominal wall are stitched one by one, with dissolving stitches. The skin will either be stitched or closed with small metal clips. It is common practice to leave a thin tube in the wound for a day or two so that excess blood and fluids can drain away. This causes little discomfort.

After the operation

Immediately after giving birth by caesarian you will be recovering in bed, usually in the postnatal ward. After a general anaesthetic, many women feel groggy and will find it difficult to focus on the baby for some time. You may be in pain, needing an injection of opiates until you are able to take ordinary pain-killing tablets. However, if you have had an epidural, pain relief can be achieved by topping up the epidural before it is removed after the birth.

You can expect to feel more comfortable within a few days of having a caesarian. Movement may be restricted for at least 24 hours by the intravenous drip providing fluids and nourishment, but you may be surprised by how soon you will be encouraged to move about. Early mobility eases breathing, improves healing and prevents blood clots developing in the leg veins.

Mother and baby usually stay in hospital for between five and ten days. The stitches or clips are removed after a week or less, and there is a postnatal checkup at six weeks. While these days many women recover remarkably quickly, it can take others between six weeks and six months before full energy returns. Plenty of rest is essential, and gentle stretching exercises started six weeks after the birth will help.

Breastfeeding your baby after a caesarian

Almost all women who have caesarians manage to breastfeed their babies. Any problems are sometimes connected with the caesarian itself - for instance, a general anaesthetic may have reached the baby and made her sleepy for a day or two - but, more often, they are linked to the reason that the caesarian was done in the first place.

Much will depend on your own optimism and determination to succeed, and on the support of those around you. It is a good idea to begin as soon as possible after the birth. The ward staff will usually encourage you, and their support will be especially important if the baby is in a special care baby unit and you are immobile for the first day or two. You will need help lifting and handling the baby, and your scar will need to be protected during feeds. To do this, you can either prop the baby up on pillows in front of you, or semi-recline on your side to feed her with a cushion between yourself and the baby to protect your abdomen.

The great benefit of breastfeeding after a caesarean is that your body produces the hormone oxytocin every time you breastfeed. This enhances bonding and the loving relationship between you and your baby.

Emotional reactions

Many mothers feel a great mixture of emotions after a caesarian. At the time, the joy and relief felt at having a baby are usually paramount. If the birth was difficult or complications arose, the caesarian is usually welcomed as the only way to a safe delivery.

However, after any major operation involving a general anaesthetic, depression is common, often on the third or fourth day. After a caesarian, this may be compounded by painful breasts, indigestion, wind and after pains. These discomforts, added to the difficulties of being physically restricted, can make the first days especially trying. You will need to rest and recuperate as well as to get to know, feed and care for your baby.

A few women feel deprived of the experience of vaginal birth, angry at having 'failed' to give birth vaginally and envious of others who have given birth normally. These feelings are entirely natural and may surface weeks or even months later. Some mothers question whether there was real need for the operation, especially if they felt pressured into having it at the time, or feel that the caesarian resulted from unnecessary intervention. Such issues are usually resolved by discussion with your attendants as soon as possible after the birth and again in the weeks that follow. The obstetrician will explain why a caesarian was the best course of action in the circumstances.

Many psychologists believe that a caesarian birth may affect a baby emotionally, especially the minority who are separated from their mothers in special care units and who will need extra love and attention. It will not matter if bonding is a little delayed as long as you are able to appreciate this special time in quiet and privacy when you are finally united with your baby. Most hospitals try to keep the separation of mothers and babies to a minimum, some allowing incubators to be placed next to the mother's bed. It may also be possible to place the baby on your chest for a while, even while being drip fed, and this will help to sustain intimacy and early bonding.

Repeat caesarean sections

Medical policy concerning subsequent births differs widely. In many parts of the United States, once a woman has had a caesarian, all her future babies will automatically be delivered in the same way, while in most other countries, this would only happen if a woman has had two caesarians.

The main concern in subsequent labours is strain on the scar in the uterus, which may tear or rupture. However, this is now very rare and, in most of Britain and Europe, each pregnancy is assessed on its own merits. Obviously if you had a caesarian because your pelvis was abnormally small, any subsequent delivery would also be a caesarian but, providing the reason for the initial operation does not recur, subsequent deliveries can usually be vaginal. You would go into labour spontaneously but with full surgical facilities on standby and the obstetrician would observe your condition, the labour, and the scar closely. This is called 'trial of scar'.

Using upright positions, or hands and knees, in such a labour is not only safe, but preferable. An active birth will usually shorten labour, help the uterus to work better and relieve pressure on the scar. In the second stage, an upright supported squat is ideal. If there are any difficulties, the obstetrician may advise a forceps or vacuum extraction. Opinions vary about labouring in a birth pool after a previous caesarian. Many practitioners feel that pressure on the abdomen is reduced under water and that this is beneficial. While labour may be in the pool the birth itself is best on dry land. Some doctors will not consider labour in water after a previous caesarian section although there is so far no evidence of any problems.

Planning Your Birth

(Creating your wish list)

Of course you cannot 'plan' your birth. This is an experience that is unknown and unpredictable. However, it is helpful to consider your options and to have a clear idea of your preferences. Creating a wish list which can be attached to your notes is an important part of your practical and emotional preparation for labour and birth. It will make communication with your birth attendants easier and encourage discussion with them and between yourselves. This will empower you to participate in the decision making about your care and to have the best possible outcome for you and your baby.

The sections below are intended as a guide to some of the possible issues you may wish to consider when creating your list. It is best to keep it fairly concise so that it is easy to read quickly and to keep an open mind about your choices so that you can respond appropriately to the circumstances at the time.

It is wise to indicate on your list that this is a guide to your preferences and that you may feel differently once you are in labour, and would like to have the freedom and flexibility to review your choices at any time.

Introduction

- **Birth partner/s**

    I will have the following person/s present with me in labour.
    Introduce yourselves, important issues, fears, concerns or special needs.
    If not your first birth, mention any relevant details about your previous experiences.

- **Place of birth**

    Home, hospital, birth centre.

- **Midwives**

    Your preference in midwife allocation, i.e. ....

    Experienced in active or water birth – willing to deliver your baby in an upright position – bed or floor!
    Is there anything your midwife should know about you?

First stage

- **Environment**

    Positioning and comfort aids
    Birth pool or bath, shower, privacy, clothes, my own music, food and drink, low lighting, beanbag or birth ball

- **Pain Relief**

    Possible options:
    Birth pool, breathing, massage, aromatherapy, homoeopathy, TENS, Entenox (gas and air), Epidural, Pethedine or Meptid

- **Monitoring and examinations**

    My preferences and requests for monitoring are:

    Pinnard (ear trumpet),
    Stethoscope,
    Hand held sonic aid,
    Waterproof sonic aid,
    Continuous monitoring on admission (CTG),
    Continuous belt monitor,
    Foetal scalp electrode or telemetry

- **Vaginal examinations**

    My feelings about these are:

- **Medical routines and interventions**

    I would like to be consulted and my consent obtained before any interventions are used.

    My feelings about the following options:
    If progress is slow:
    - First try position change, increased privacy, aromatherapy, homoeopathy.

    If induced:
    - Prostaglandin gel or pessary / or other drugs used to ripen the cervix
    - Breaking waters to initiate labour / to accelerate labour
    - Syntocinon drip to initiate labour / to accelerate labour.

Transition

- **Environment** — Privacy, darkness, quiet, minimum disturbance, warmth.

- **Pain Relief** — Non medical, medical (i.e. entenox).

- **Examinations** — Avoid routine vaginal exam, minimal disturbance.

Second stage

- Positions I might like to use in second stage

- My feelings about pushing in second stage

- In the event of an assisted birth my feelings are:

    (i.e. episiotomy, ventouse, forceps, caesarean section)

- My preferences for anaesthesia for instrumental delivery or caesarean

    (i.e. epidural, spinal, general anaesthetic)

- My feelings about hands off or poised as the babies head emerges

Third stage

- Environment

  Privacy, warmth, no disturbance

- Physiological third stage

  I would like my baby to be given to me immediately if possible.
  I do / do not want to be told the baby's sex; I would like to start breastfeeding right away if possible.

- Syntometrine

  My preferences are:
  Routinely administered; after the cord stops pulsating; not at all unless heavy bleeding; after placenta is expelled, only if medically necessary or if birth was induced or accelerated.

- Cutting and clamping the umbilical cord

  immediately (eg after syntometrine), after pulsation ceases, after the placenta is expelled.

After the birth

- Sensitive handling of the baby
- If I have a general anaesthetic
- Suctioning
- Examinations of the newborn including preferences for administration of vitamin K
- Feeding preferences
- Discharge from hospital.

Any further comments, preferences or concerns

Student midwives and doctors involved in your care

Any special concerns, other...

It is advisable to discuss your wish list with your midwives and to keep a copy in your notes which you have signed and a midwife or doctor at the antenatal clinic has signed. To aid communication, show your wish list to each midwife who attends your labour.

Notes

Active Birth Manifesto

1. In every uninhibited labour there is a marked restlessness: the woman walks, stands, squats, kneels, lies down and moves her body freely to find the most comfortable and appropriate positions. There can be no fixed position for a natural healthy labour and birth when a woman follows her own instincts - for birth is active, involving a succession of changing positions and is not a passive confinement.

2. Throughout the world, and for thousands of years, women have spontaneously laboured and given birth in some form of upright or crouching positions - often supported. Whatever the race or culture: African, American, Asian, European and so on, the same upright positions predominate. History confirms the evidence of ethnologists showing the prevalent use of vertical positions throughout the ages.

3. Most women in post industrialised countries today are confined in a recumbent or semi-recumbent position, usually in hospital. This practice is illogical, making birth needlessly complicated and expensive, turning a natural process into a medical event and the labouring woman into a passive patient. No other species adopts such a disadvantageous position at such a crucial time.

4. Research reveals serious disadvantages to the use of the recumbent position:

- Lying on the back causes compression of the major abdominal blood vessels along the spinal column. Compression of the large artery of the heart (descending aorta) hinders circulation to the uterus and placenta and can result in foetal distress. Compression of the large veins leading to the heart (inferior vena cava) restricts the returning blood flow and can contribute to hypotension and other circulatory problems, increasing the risk of heavy bleeding after birth.

- The recumbent position reduces the potential mobility of the pelvic joints, in particular the advantages of flexing the knees and hips in an upright posture, i.e. the acute angle made by bringing the knees towards the chest (as in squatting) which opens and widens the pelvis to its maximum. In the reclining position the body weight rests directly on the sacrum and prevents the pivotal movement of the posterior wall of the pelvis to accommodate the baby's descending head. This significantly reduces the diameter of the pelvic outlet between the symphysis pubis and the coccyx, losing up to 30 percent of the potential opening, compared with squatting or leaning forward.

- It is easier for an object to fall towards the earth's surface than to slide parallel to it (Newton's law of gravity). In reclining positions the uterus has to work in opposition to gravity. This wastes energy, causes unnecessary effort and pain

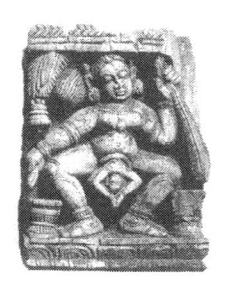

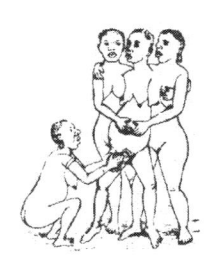

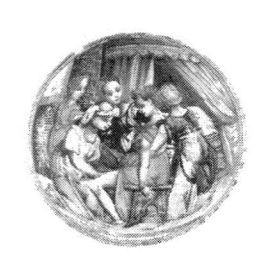

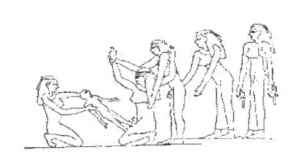

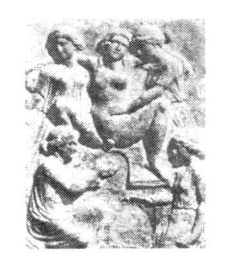

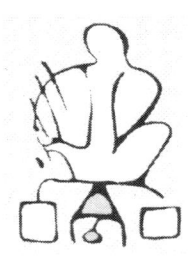

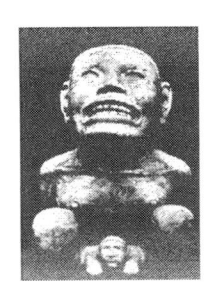

© Janet Balaskas 2001

while increasing the duration of labour and birth. The descent, rotation and birth of the baby are made easier when the maternal position directs the baby towards the earth rather than along the horizon.

- Malpresentations are more likely when the spontaneous movements of the mother which guide the baby's rotation through the birth canal are restricted.

- When lying down for the birth, the perineal tissues stretch unevenly at the expense of the posterior part, this causes stress and pain and increases the risk of tearing or the need for episiotomy.

5. Movement and position change is more important than a single optimal or best position during labour. Spontaneous labour positions include standing, walking, sitting upright, kneeling, crouching or resting on one side.

A labour position is physiologically effective when:
- there is no compression on the blood vessels
- movement is unrestricted
- the pelvis is fully mobilised
- the body works in harmony with gravity

For birth, squatting and its variants are the positions closest to nature's laws and are known as physiological birth positions. These include full or semi squats, standing squats or various kneeling positions.

The use of such upright positions produce the following additional benefits in the second stage:
- more powerful contractions resulting in an effective expulsive reflex
- optimal foetal oxygenation
- minimal strain and muscular effort
- an optimal angle of descent
- maximum space for descent, rotation and emergence of the presenting parts through the pelvic outlet.
- optimal relaxation of the perineum.

It has been demonstrated that where the use of upright positions during labour and birth is actively encouraged, the number of spontaneous physiological births increases.

6. In an active birth the physiological process unfolds spontaneously due to the uninhibited release of birth hormones. Oxytocin secretion is optimal, resulting in efficient contractions in labour, an effective expulsive reflex during birth, expedient delivery of the placenta and good retraction of the uterus thereafter. High endorphine levels increase the mother's ability to cope with pain without intervention. The altruistic effects of the high hormone levels in both mother and baby promote normal attachment and bonding in the critical first hour after birth.

7. The importance of a conducive environment for labour and birth, where the mother feels safe and secure and where her privacy is protected, is of paramount

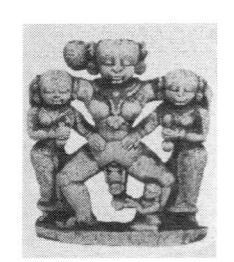

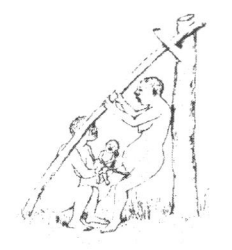

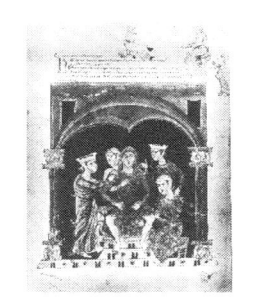

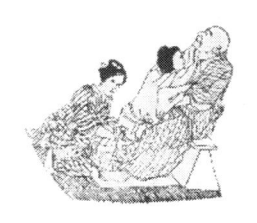

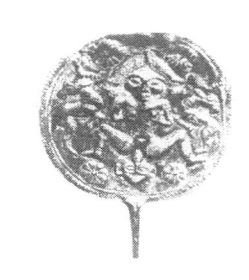

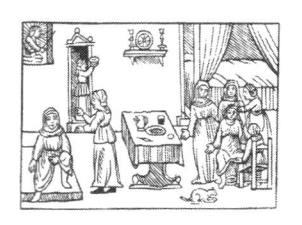

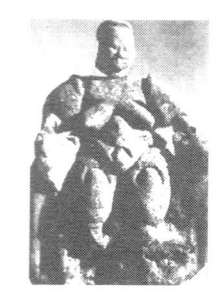

© Janet Balaskas 2001

importance. Such conditions are essential to ensure spontaneous movement in upright positions and also for optimal hormone secretion - the key features of an active birth.

8. Immersion in warm water at approximately body temperature in the active stage of labour (5-6 cms dilation) has been shown to enhance an active birth. Contractions may intensify and the buoyancy increases relaxation, comfort and mobility. Studies have shown that pain modification is significant. While primarily intended to ease labour, a birthing pool can also provide a suitable environment for the birth, when conditions are optimal.

9. Numerous studies in the last 50 years indicate that when birth is active the advantages are:
- the natural rhythm and continuity of birth are not disrupted.
- uterine contractions are stronger, more regular and more frequent.
- dilation is enhanced.
- more complete relaxation is possible between contractions.
- intrauterine pressure is consistently higher.
- first and second stages of labour are shorter - some studies show over 40 percent shorter in the upright group.
- there is greater comfort, less stress and pain, so decreased need for analgesia.
- the condition of the newborn is generally optimal.
- women feel that they are fully participating, in control and more often experience giving birth as a wonderful and joyous experience.

10. There is no doubt to anyone who has experienced or witnessed both active and passive birth, that an active labour and birth is usually easier, safer and more rewarding for both mother and child. After an active birth, the mother feels that she has given birth, rather than having had her baby extracted from her. She and her baby have been full participants together and both are alert, undrugged and healthy when they meet face to face. This inevitably results in the best possible conditions for maternal/infant attachment and the foundation of healthy loving relationships in the family.

11. Active birth is more than a matter of positions. While the freedom to move spontaneously and to use upright positions is fundamental, the essential definition of an active birth is one in which the birthing mother is in charge of her choices and decisions. This enables her to enjoy a productive and mutually respectful partnership with her birth attendants. When interventions are necessary, the principles of an active birth may still be useful in combination with obstetric procedures, and help to minimise risks or side effects. When this is the case, every birth, whether natural or assisted, may be called an active birth.

12. The long term consequences of unnecessary intervention around the time of birth to health and well being is an area of increasing concern. Based on research findings, modern experience and ancestral instinct, fundamental changes in attitude and provision of maternity services, in the education of midwives and in the

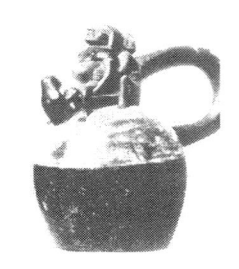

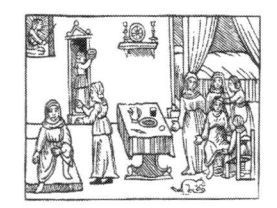

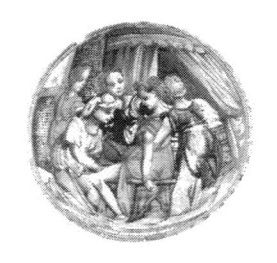

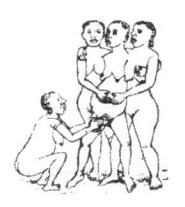

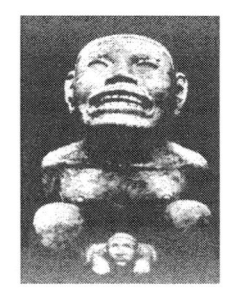

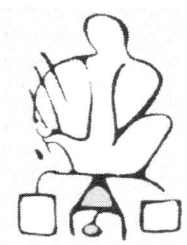

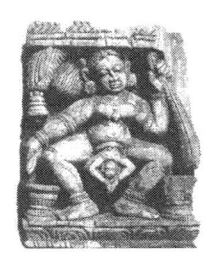

© Janet Balaskas 2001

preparation of women for birth are inevitable, in order to increase the potential for physiological birth.

13. Childbirth, in any woman's life, is an exceptional act, a tour de force, partly instinctive and partly a learned skill. There is a knack to doing most things and birth is no exception. A prospective mother needs more than knowledge and information about pregnancy, labour and birth. She also needs physical, mental and emotional preparation throughout pregnancy, to develop comfort and ease in upright positions and confidence in her innate ability to give birth. Preparation for an active birth needs to offer her a means of profound and deep relaxation of body and mind, to enable her to access and trust her instinctual potential.

14. As well as a celebration in the family, the birth of a child is a critical, uncertain event involving suspense as to the final outcome. The skill of birth giving and of birth attendance is prized in every society. In the modern and western world, the application of technology to birth has introduced unprecedented safety and lifesaving procedures. However, the widespread and routine application of such technologies to the majority of women is inappropriate and has been demonstrated to increase the number of complicated and surgical births all over the world. This leads to the loss of valuable and essential midwifery skills and increasing reliance on technology, eroding the satisfaction and confidence of both mothers and midwives. Medical attendants have become the birth experts. Moreover, the balance of power is such that the skill of the birthing woman has been so undermined, that most women have lost touch with the age-old knowledge and wisdom of birthing that was previously handed down the generations, mother to mother. This balance of skill and power must be restored by reclaiming the instinctive potential, freedom and power of the giver of birth, the mother. The Active Birth Movement is committed to the empowerment of birthing women and the global rediscovery of birth.

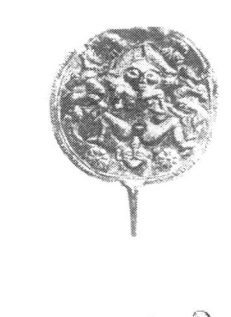

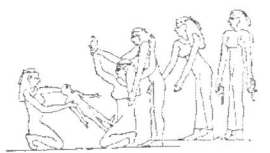

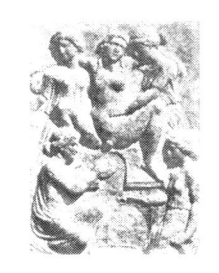

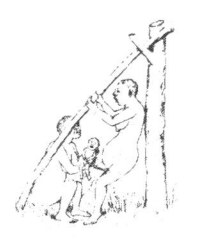

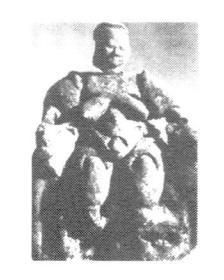

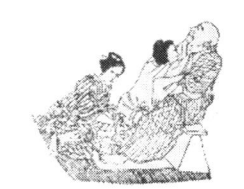

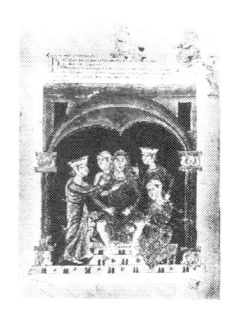

First written in April 1982 by Janet and Arthur Balaskas
Revised by Janet Balaskas in February 2001

© Copyright Janet Balaskas 2001
No part of the above text may be reproduced in any form
whatsoever without prior permission from Janet Balaskas.

Bibliography

Books and reports

Arms, S. *Immaculate Deception II - Myth, Magic and Birth.* Celestial Arts. 1994
Balaskas, J. *Active Birth.* Thorsons UK, Harvard Common Press. US 1992
Beech, B. *Water Birth Unplugged.* Books for Midwives 1996
Burns, E., Kitzinger, S. *Midwifery Guidelines for Use of Water in Labour.* Oxford Brookes University. 2000
Enkin, M., et al. *A Guide to Effective Care in Pregnancy and Childbirth.* 3rd Edition. Oxford University Press. 2000
Flint, C. *Sensitive Midwifery.* Butterworth Heinemann. 1986
Francome C, Savage W, et al. *Caesarean Birth in Britain.* Middlesex University Press. 1993
Gelis, J. *History of Childbirth - Fertility, Pregnancy and Birth in Early Modern Europe.* Polity Press. 1991
Goer, H. *Obstetric Myths versus Research Realities: A Guide to the medical literature.* Bergin & Garvey. USA 1995
Odent, M. *The Nature of Birth and Breastfeeding.* Bergin and Harvey. 1992
Odent, M. *Birth Reborn.* Souvenir Press: 2nd edition. London 1994
Odent, M. *The Scientification of Love.* Free Association Books. London 1999
Prija, J.V. *Birth Traditions and Modern Pregnancy Care.* Element Books. 1992
Robertson, A. *Empowering Women.* ACE Graphics. 1994
Simkin, P. and Ancheta, R. *The labor progress handbook.* Blackwell Science. Oxford 2000
Tew, M. *Safer Childbirth? A Critical History of Maternity Care.* Chapman and Hall. 1990
Thomas, P. *Every Woman's Birth Rights.* Thorsons. 1996
Wagner, M. *Pursuing the Birth Machine - The search for Appropriate Birth Technology.* ACE Graphics. 1994
Report of the Expert Maternity Group. *Changing Childbirth.* HMSO. 1994
Winterton Report 1992. *The House of Commons Health Committee 2nd Report.* Maternity Services Vol.1 HMSO 1992

Articles

1. Arroyo. J., Menendez, A., Salmean, J., Manas, J., Lavilla, M., Martin, S.M., Elizaga, I.V., Crespo, J.Z. *Effects of different positions in labour.* Fifth European Congress of Perinatal Medicine, Sweden 1976

2. Caldeyro-Bacia, R. *The influence of maternal position on time of spontaneous rupture of the membranes, progress of labour, and foetal head compression.* Birth and Family. Journal 6:1, 1979. pp.7-15

3. Broadhurst, A, Flynn, A M, Kelly, J and others. *The effects of ambulation in labour on maternal satisfaction, analgesia and lactation.* In: Zichella (ed) Proceedings of the 5th International Congress of Psychosomatic Medicine in Obstetrics and Gynecology, Rome, 1979, pp 943-946

4. Chan, D.C.P. *Positions in labour.* British Medical Journal. 1:12, 1963 pp.100-102

5. Clarke, A.P. *The influence of position of the patient in labour in causing uterine inertia and pelvic disturbances.* Journal of American Medical Association 16, 1891. pp.433-435

7. Diaz, A.G., Schqarez, R., Fescina, Y.R., Caldeyro-Barcia, R *Efectos de la position vertical materna sobre la evolution del parto.* Separata de la Revista Clinica e Investigation en Ginecologia y Obstetrica, 3. 1978. pp.101-109

8. Flynn, A.M., Kelly, J., Hollins, G. and others. *Ambulation in labour.* British Medical Journal. 2:26, 1978, pp.591-593

9. Gardosi, J., Sylvester, S. and B-Lynch, G. *Alternative positions in the Second Stage of labour; a randomised trial.* British Journal of Obstetrics and Gynaecology 1996: 1290-96. 1989

10. Gestaldo, T.D. *The Significance of maternal position on pelvic outlet dimensions.* Correspondence, Birth 19. 14: 230. 1992

11. Gupta, J.K., Nikodem, C. *Maternal posture in labour.* European Journal of Obstetrics and Gynaecology and Reproductive Biology. 92:2, 2000. pp. 273-277

12. Haire, D. *Obstetric drugs and procedures: Their effects on mother and baby. (Part 1)* AIMS (Australia) Quarterly Journal 6. 1: 1-8. 1994

13. Humphrey, M., Hunslow, D., Morgan, S., Wood, C. *The influence of maternal posture at birth on the foetus.* Journal of Obstetrics and Gynaecology. British Commonwealth 80. 1973 pp. 1075-1080

14. De Jong, P.R., Johanson, R.B., Blaxen, P. and others. *Randomised trial comparing the upright and supine positions for the second stage of labour.* British Journal of Obstetrics and Gynaecology, 104:5 1997 pp. 567-571

15. Joseph, J. *The joints of the pelvis and their relation to posture in labour.* Midwives Chronicle, 101:1202, 1988. pp. 63-64
16. Kimball, C.D., Chang, C.M. et al. *Immunoreactive endorphin peptides and prolactin in umbilical vein and maternal blood.* American Journal of Obstetrics and Gynaecology. 14:104-5; 1987
17. King, A.F.A. *The significance of posture in obstetrics.* New York Medical Journal 80, 1909 pp.1054-1058
18. Kouvenen, K., Teramo, K. *Effects of maternal position on fetal heart during extradural analgesia.* British Journal of Anaesthesia 51:767, 1979.
19. Liu, Y.C. *The effects of the upright position during childbirth.* Image: Journal of Nursing Scholarship, 21:1, 1989. pp. 14-18
20. Markoe, J.W. *Posture in obstetrics. Bulletin Lying in Hospital.* NY 11. 1917 pp.11-26
21. McKay, S., Roberts, J. *Second stage labour: what is normal?* Journal of Obstetric, Gynecologic, and Neonatal Nursing, 14:2 1985. pp.101-108
22. McKay, S. *Squatting: an alternate position for the second stage of labour.* MCN- American Journal of Maternal/Child Nursing, 9, May/June 1984 pp.181-183
23. McManus, T.J., Calder, A.A. *Upright posture and the efficiency of labour.* Lancet 1:14 1978 pp.72-74
24. Mendez-Bauer, C., Arroyo, J., Zamarriego, J.O. *Maternal standing position in first stage of labour.* Reviews in Perinatal Medicine. Vol 1, Eds Scarpelli, E.M. and Cosmi, E.V. Baltimore, University Park Press 1976. pp. 281-293
25. Mitre, N. *The influence of maternal position on duration of the active phase of labour.* International Journal of Gynaecology and Obstetrics, 12:5 1974 pp.181-183
26. Moss, I. R., Conner, H. et al. *Human beta endorphin-like immuno-reactivity in the perinatal/neonatal period.* Journal of Pediatrics. 1982. 101; 3:443-46.
27. Newton, N. *The fetus ejection reflex revisited.* Birth 1987; 14:106-8
28. Nikodem, V.C. *Immersion in water during pregnancy, labour and birth.* (Most recent amendment, June 1997). The Cochrane Library, Oxford - 1998, Issue 1.
29. Odent, M. *Birth under Water.* Lancet. Dec 24 1983. pp.1476-77
30. Odent, M. *Position in delivery.* Lancet. May 12 1990. p.1166
31. Odent, M. *The fetus ejection reflex.* Birth. 1987. 14:104-5
32. Read, J.A., Miller, F.C., and Paul, R.H. (1981) *Ambulation versus oxytocin for labour enhancement.* American Journal of Obstetrics and Gynaecology 139:669-72.
33. Rhodes, P. *Posture in obstetrics.* Physiotherapy 1967 53: pp.158-163
34. Roberts, J.E. *Maternal positions for childbirth: a historical review of nursing care practices.* Journal of Obstetric, Gynaecologic and Neonatal Nursing, 8, Jan/Feb 1979 pp.24-32
35. Roberts, J.E. *Alternative frontiers for childbirth.* Journal of Nurse Midwifery. 25:4 1980
36. Roberts, J.E., Mendez-Bauer, C., Wodell, D.A. *The effects of maternal position on uterine contractility and efficiency.* Birth, 10:4, 1983. pp.243-249
37. Simpkin, P. (1991/2) *Just another day in a woman's life? Women's long term perceptions of their first birth experience.* Parts 1 and 2, Birth 18.4: 203-10; and Birth 19.2: 64-81
38. *Stand and deliver.* Lancet, 335:8692, 1990 pp.761-762
39. Stewart, P., Spiby, H. *Posture in labour.* British Journal of Obstetrics & Gynaecology, 96:11, 1989, pp.1258-1260
40. Stewart, P. *Influence of posture in labour.* Contemporary Reviews in Obstetrics and Gynaecology, 3:3 1991 pp.152-157
41. Stewart, P., Calder, A.A. *Posture in Labour: patients' choice and its effect on performance.* British Journal of Obstetrics and Gynaecology, 91:11 1984 pp.1091-1095
42. Taffel, S. M., Placek, P. J. and Kosary, C. L. (1992) *U.S caesarean section rates 1990: An update.* Birth, Vol.19, no. 1, pp.21-2
43. Tew, M. (1986) *Do obstetric intranatal interventions make birth safer?* British Journal of Obstetrics and Gynaecology 93: 659-74
44. Walsh, D. *Birth positions in a large consultant unit.* The Practising Midwife, June 1998 Vol. 1 No 6, pp 34-35
45. Williams, R.M., Thom, M., Studd, J.W.W. *A study of the benefits and acceptability of ambulation in spontaneous labour.* British Journal of Obstetrics and Gynaecology, 87:2 1980 pp. 122-126

Made in the USA
Columbia, SC
06 March 2018